999

MY LIFE ON THE FRONTLINE
OF THE AMBULANCE SERVICE

DAN FARNWORTH

WITH BENJAMIN DIRS

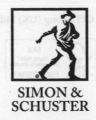

**SIMON &
SCHUSTER**

London · New York · Sydney · Toronto · New Delhi

First published in Great Britain by Simon & Schuster UK Ltd, 2020
This edition published in Great Britain by Simon & Schuster UK Ltd, 2021

Copyright © Dan Farnworth, 2020

The right of Dan Farnworth to be identified as the author
of this work has been asserted in accordance with the
Copyright, Designs and Patents Act, 1988.

1 3 5 7 9 10 8 6 4 2

Simon & Schuster UK Ltd
1st Floor
222 Gray's Inn Road
London WC1X 8HB

www.simonandschuster.co.uk
www.simonandschuster.com.au
www.simonandschuster.co.in

Simon & Schuster Australia, Sydney
Simon & Schuster India, New Delhi

A CIP catalogue record for this book is available from the British Library

Paperback ISBN: 978-1-4711-8444-4
eBook ISBN: 978-1-4711-8443-7

For Maddison, Rhianna, Courtney and Harrison.
And for Mum and Dad – my beacons in the toughest
times, who helped make me the person I am today.

In memory of Paul Edmondson, a true legend
and an amazing son, father, brother and friend.

CONTENTS

AUTHOR'S NOTE

Although I have not identified people and places, for reasons of privacy, the events in this book are described as happened. I wrote this book for a few main reasons: first, so that the public might have a better understanding of what an ambulance person's job entails; second, as a tribute to my colleagues, who continue to work wonders in difficult circumstances, and to the NHS, which is undoubtedly creaking, but remains a beacon of hope for so many; and third, to highlight the strain the job puts on an ambulance person's mental health and my efforts to raise awareness of this problem.

PROLOGUE: ALL WE CAN DO

It was a dark and stormy night. The rain fell in torrents . . .

Actually, that's a big, fat fib. It's never that dramatic and there are rarely any omens. The night in question – as with most nights in the ambulance service – was like any other bog-standard midweek shift. We may have attended an elderly woman who had fallen over on her way to the toilet and a middle-aged man who had woken up with chest pains. What you might call our bread and butter. Did a drunk bloke try to punch me? Maybe. It's happened more than once. There was hardly any traffic on the roads and more foxes than people on the pavements. Which was preferable, as foxes have the good grace and manners not to get bladdered on Jägerbombs and collapse in shop doorways.

We get a call from the police: 'We've got this guy on the phone, telling us he's killed his mum with an axe. Thing is, he's always saying this. Either he had ten mums or he's making it up again. Will you go and have a look?'

Just to confirm: the police want us to attend a patient who's claiming he's killed his mum with an axe, even though we don't have weapons, stab vests or any training in dealing with the mentally ill? This could be interesting.

I turn to my partner and say, 'Sod this, unless they provide us with full suits of body armour, I ain't going in without the police.'

The bloke is most likely talking a load of nonsense, but what if this is the one time he's telling the truth? I've got four kids, for God's sake.

So we drive to the address, at the most undramatic speed imaginable, park up around the corner from the axe murderer's house and stake the place out. But staking places out is a bit difficult in an ambulance: I don't know if you've noticed, but they're custard yellow with a flashing blue light on the top.

Me and my partner spend the next forty minutes swapping tales of dramatic and traumatic jobs, before the police finally turn up. Thanks for popping in, lads.

We line up behind two coppers on the axe murderer's doorstep, the door swings open and there he is in all his drunken glory, staggering all over his hallway and telling us to piss off. In the strongest terms, he denies making any phone calls, and while he's doing so, his cat escapes. Now he's telling us that he used to be in the Royal Marines and that if we don't find his cat, he'll beat us all up. The police's reaction? 'Can we go now?' Our reaction? 'Can we come in and assess you?' His reaction? 'Clear off, ya bastards!'

This is a bit of a dilemma. If we leave without assessing him and he falls down the stairs, the fact he's told us to leave him alone is neither here nor there. But what can you do when you're faced with an aggressive ex-Marine-cum-axe murderer? The police have a quick look around his house, find no sign of a dead mum and get the hell out of Dodge. We're right behind them.

Back in the ambulance, a new job appears on our screen: SEVEN-WEEK-OLD CHILD, NOT BREATHING. CARDIAC ARREST. My heart sinks. This is every ambulance person's worst nightmare. I switch on the blue lights and floor it.

It's not uncommon to be told a child is not breathing, only to arrive at the job to find a panicky mum and a toddler with some mucus stuck in his throat. I don't blame the parents; it must be terrifying. But sometimes you just have a bad feeling in the pit of your stomach. You might call it an ambulance person's sixth sense, the ability to predict whether an emergency is genuine.

This job is just around the corner from the hospital, so we have a decision to make. The hospital has doctors, nurses, paediatricians and a hundred other specialists, while our ambulance contains an emergency medical technician – i.e. me – and a paramedic, who in this case is fairly new to the job. If we were miles away from the hospital, we'd stay in the house, administer the drugs and try to do everything in our power to resuscitate the child before whisking it away. But on this occasion, we have a quick chat and decide to get to the house, pick up the baby and leg it, as fast as our ambulance will carry us. In the trade, we call it a 'scoop and run'. As is often the case in the ambulance service, it's a cheery phrase that belies its seriousness.

We can only drive an ambulance 20mph over the limit, and it's not a rule that's usually flouted. There's no point in driving so fast that you crash into a wall and never make it. I call it 'driving to arrive'. And it doesn't matter if you're on your way to a family stuck in a house fire or a car wreck, if you run someone over and they die, you will end up in court. But this particular job is a case of bollocks to the rules.

We pull up outside the house, jump out of the ambulance and can hear a woman screaming, 'My baby! My baby!'

And it suddenly hits me, like a breeze block to the face: this is it, the job we train for. If an elderly woman falling on her way to the toilet is a league fixture, this is a cup final. I have to be at the top of my game. I have to do things right, because there is so much at stake. I jump in the back of the ambulance and grab everything we might need: the defibrillator, an ALS (advanced life support) bag, oxygen, drugs and a bag of other tricks. Unfortunately, the bag of tricks doesn't contain a magic wand.

We march through the open front door looking like a couple of packhorses – equipment and bags hanging over shoulders, round necks and off every finger and thumb – and head in the direction of the screaming. As I climb the stairs, the adrenalin kicks in and everything starts moving in slow motion, which means I'm able to process things faster. I repeat to myself, 'ABC – airway, breathing, circulation. Just do what you've been taught.'

We walk into the main bedroom to find the baby on the floor, with its dad attempting CPR (cardiopulmonary resuscitation). The baby is seven weeks old. It is white, floppy and bleeding from the nose. In short, it looks like the odds are stacked against it.

We shoo the dad aside and try to do what we can. A child will normally stop breathing because of an airway obstruction, so we try to oxygenate it and apply compressions to the chest to get the circulation going. Instead of doing it with two hands and jumping up and down, like you would with an adult, I lightly press with two fingers. But I don't even bother opening my bag of tricks. Instead, I go straight to the radio on my hip and call the hospital: 'Red pre-alert. We're coming in with a child. Seven weeks old. In cardiac arrest. You've got sixty seconds to get ready.'

My partner grabs the baby, I grab the bags, we run to the ambulance, bundle Mum and Dad into the back and get going. While I'm tear-arsing it to the hospital, my partner is battling to save the baby's life in the back, which is like trying to thread a needle at sea in a storm.

From arriving at the house to arriving at the hospital takes no more than three minutes, so I kind of expect them not to be ready. Ambulance people are cynical like that, but for good reason. It's not uncommon to arrive at the hospital and find people queuing out of the doors, which means we have to wait with our patients while they deal with other emergencies. As harsh as it sounds, there is a pecking order. If you go to hospital with a broken arm, you might have to wait for hours. Even if you're having a heart attack, you might have to wait ten minutes while they deal with something more pressing. And there is almost always something more pressing. But on this occasion, the staff are waiting like coiled springs. What happens next is incredible to witness.

I place the baby on a bed and continue ventilating before the specialists take over. An anaesthetist sweeps in, along with paediatricians, who intubate the baby (put a tube down its throat to assist breathing). There must be between fifteen and twenty medical professionals working on the patient, including me, passing bits and bobs to the doctors. Being part of that process is like being part of a magnificent machine, each component working in perfect harmony.

The whole time we're working, we can hear the baby's mum screaming, 'My baby! My baby! Why won't she open her eyes?' and her dad muttering, over and over again, 'It's all my fault . . .'

The story of how the baby came to be in our care follows in snippets. The dad had fallen asleep on his bed next to the baby, rolled over and suffocated it. Maybe that explained the bleeding nose. Meanwhile, the poor mum had been out with friends for the first time since her baby was born. Imagine that, popping out for a couple of drinks and a catch-up, before coming back a few hours later to a baby that was seemingly dead. He blames himself, she blames herself, maybe they both blame each other. I turn to see the dad on the floor, curled up into a ball, next to the mum, sobbing uncontrollably. By being in the room, at least they know we're doing everything we can. How much that will help is up for debate.

After almost an hour of non-stop treatment, the decision is made to cease CPR. The mum screams again, 'No! You can't stop!' But the baby is dead, so there is nothing more we can do. A nurse dresses the baby in a babygro, places it in a Moses basket and puts it in a quiet room where Mum and Dad can say their goodbyes. I'm not sure you could imagine a more tragic scene. As I slip away, I can't help wondering what life has in store for that poor couple. Will they ever get over it? Will they ever make peace with each other? Will they ever have another baby? If so, will it rid them of the pain?

———

Ambulance people come barging into people's lives at the most critical moments, do what they can do, then disappear into the ether. I'll often pick up little bits of the backstory, usually from a friend or a family member. Or, at least, their interpretation of it. But more often than not, I'll turn up at the house of someone who's had a cardiac arrest, for example, put them in the ambulance, take them to hospital, head to the next job and never find out if they survived or not.

Occasionally, curiosity will get the better of me and I'll phone the hospital and say, 'Hi, I was with the ambulance crew that brought in so and so. Could you tell me how he is?' And the nurse will almost always tell me that they can't, because of patient confidentiality. Unless the story is newsworthy enough to make the papers or appear on the internet, we never find out. That means we're able to tell an awful lot of dramatic stories with no neat resolutions. That can be frustrating but is probably for the best. Ambulance people invest enough emotion in their jobs as it is. Learning that a patient I fought tooth and nail to save didn't pull through is unlikely to make me sleep any easier.

Nevertheless, the story of how we tried to save that baby's life illustrates a powerful point: all those articles you've read in the newspapers about the ambulance service and the whole NHS being at melting point are true. But when things go really pear-shaped, we pull out all the stops. I honestly believe our paramedics and technicians are the finest in the world, and the doctors in our hospitals are trained to within an inch of their lives. That baby might only have been seven weeks old, but it had hundreds of years of expertise trying to save its life.

In my fifteen years on the frontline, I've seen so many lives lost, but so many lives saved. Either way, and despite all the obstacles strewn in our path, we've always given it our best and I've never stopped being enormously proud.

Unfortunately, pride isn't a salve for what we witness. Ambulance people work themselves to their absolute limit. We graft for hours on end with very few breaks so that we're there when your mum falls over and breaks her hip; your dad has a stroke; your son falls out of a tree and fractures his skull; your partner takes an overdose. And they're just the regulation jobs. Some of the other stuff we deal with would be considered too graphic to make the final cut of a particularly horrifying horror film. And after we've done what we can do to make things better, we put what we've witnessed in a mental filing cabinet, kick the door closed and head straight to the next job.

While we always do everything we can possibly do to help, it sometimes feels that nobody is there to help us. Knowing that I work for an institution as beloved as the NHS is a comfort. But not as much as someone simply saying, 'How are you feeling?'

1

ONE IN, ONE OUT

I often get kids coming up to me and saying, 'I want to be an ambulance person. Is it a good job?' If I've just had a bad day I might reply, 'Maybe have a look at being a train driver first. You can earn a lot more money and it's a lot less stressful. Or if you're any good at football, give that a try instead.' But if I'm in a better mood I'll say, 'If that's what you really want to do, give it a crack. Being an ambulance person is better than sitting behind a desk all day.'

I work with people who are clever enough to be bankers, insurance brokers or businesspeople. They could have opted for working in an office earning 100 grand a year instead of working in the ambulance service, resuscitating the dying, taking away the dead and not getting paid a great deal for it. But would their life be as fulfilling? Probably not. NHS staff, from well-paid consultants down to those earning not much more than the minimum wage, just want to help people. That's a good way to spend a working life. At least when I finally hang up my defibrillator, I'll be able to say, 'I didn't make much money, but at least I was working for the greater good of humanity.'

People sometimes ask me what a normal day consists of in the ambulance service. There is no normal day. But, believe it or not, the job can be quite routine. We try to arrive at the station fifteen to twenty minutes before the start of our shift so that we can grab a cuppa and the previous crew can knock off early (although they'll often still be out on a job). If there is a crew waiting, we'll grab the keys and radios from them, open up the ambulance and make sure everything is ship-shape and Bristol fashion. Have we got all the drugs we might need? Are they all in date? Do we have splints and bandages, an oxygen mask, a stretcher? It's not cool for a crew to leave an ambulance in a ramshackle state – when you hand over the keys, it should be ready for the next crew to jump in and go. That said, if they've had a really rough shift, they might leave a note saying, 'We've cleaned it, but you might need to stock up on a few things.'

I know I might not have a break for six to eight hours, so I'll stash a sweaty sandwich in the door pocket, before turning on my radio, logging on to the dashboard computer and waiting for the first job to come in – which usually takes less than a minute. An address will appear on the screen and off we'll pop, automatically guided by a very clever satnav. If the call has been waiting a while, we'll get all the information straightaway: ELDERLY MAN, FITTING. If not, we're drip-fed updates on the way, depending on what questions the call-taker has asked and what answers have been provided by the caller. We'll also be provided with a category of seriousness, more on which later.

Every gig is different, because every person is different. But different bodies still go wrong in the same way. We deal with a lot of people with chest and back pain, shortness of breath, cuts, bumps, bruises and breaks. After a while, applying a particular set of solutions to a particular set of problems becomes second nature. I wouldn't say being an ambulance person ever gets boring, but it can be quite samey.

There are days when I wake up and think, *I hope nothing big happens today*, because I've had a bad night's sleep or I'm just not feeling too chipper. But thinking like that is tempting fate. An ambulance person can never allow themselves to become complacent. It's not as if we can go out and get hammered, drag ourselves out of bed the following morning, turn up late and breathe whisky fumes over some poor old girl who's taken a tumble. Even seemingly 'normal' days in the ambulance service – which you might define as any day when nothing happens that makes you despair of the world – can turn into horror shows in the time it takes to say, 'Shit, there's been a major traffic accident on the M40 . . .'

But I'd be lying if I said ambulance people don't relish the different and the dramatic, because it challenges us to think outside the box and tests our training to its limits. There is something thrilling about doing a job that can chuck something new at you at any moment. I might spend eight hours on a shift dealing with coughs and colds, and then suddenly something comes in which has me sitting bolt upright in the ambulance thinking, *I really need to have my wits about me for this next one.* A child might have had an anaphylaxis – which is a severe allergic reaction – and will require the administration of a bucketload of drugs. Or someone might have jumped off the third floor of a multistorey car park and suffered traumatic injuries. At times like those, we need to be on our game.

———

It was Christmas Day, although I can't remember which year. It all tends to merge into one.

A call comes on our screen: ELDERLY LADY STOPPED BREATHING. I put my foot down and we're at the scene before you can say 'may your days be merry and bright'. All the family are round for turkey dinner, wearing Christmas jumpers and paper hats. I ask where the patient is and her son leads us into a bedroom. As soon as I see her, flat on her back on the floor, I know she's dead. It's rare for anyone to go into cardiac arrest out of hospital and survive. We administer CPR, give drugs and intubate, to no avail. Normally if someone dies at home, we leave them for a private ambulance to come and take them to a place of rest, but it doesn't feel right leaving that lady on the floor on Christmas Day. So we put her on a stretcher, place her in the back of the ambulance and take her to hospital. One job down, how many more to go?

Next up, a childbirth. One out, one in, like some cosmic nightclub. When me and my partner arrive, a lady is sat on her living room floor, next to her partner. The baby's head is already on its way out. 'Hello,' I say, 'my name's Dan.' I don't need to ask her what the problem is.

I'm not a big fan of childbirth jobs. For starters, it's just quite an awkward, invasive situation. It's the first time you've ever met and she's lying on the floor with her legs akimbo. It's also not nice seeing someone in so much pain. The smell is sickly sweet and, when you're crouched at the business end, it's certainly not a sight for the squeamish. Not only that, an ambulance person can go months or even years without delivering a baby, which means we can get rusty. It's not as if we can practise, like footballers practise penalties or golfers practise bunker shots. People say that delivering a baby is like riding a bike, but it isn't. We forget

15

things. But we can't use that as an excuse for not delivering a baby safely.

Childbirths are unpredictable, which makes them stressful. There are a million and one things to do, and they all need doing now. But we still need to do them in a measured, methodical way. An ambulance person is not really in control of a childbirth, the mother is. We're just a coach, telling her to breathe and push at the right times. And when the deed is done, there are suddenly two patients: a mother who might be bleeding heavily and a baby who is at risk of all sorts of complications. All of the above is why we have midwives. Unfortunately, midwives don't have blue lights and sirens.

The key to keeping a patient calm, regardless of how uncertain we are about a situation, is appearing calm ourselves. If we can appear calm on the surface, however frantically we're paddling underneath, we'll be able to keep control of things. With this in mind, never play an ambulance person at poker.

Another reason you'll also hardly ever see an ambulance crew running into a house is that treating a patient, especially administering CPR or delivering a baby, can be bloody hard work. There's no point huffing and puffing all over a patient when you're supposed to be there to help them. So we usually go in slow and weigh up the scene, which can sometimes look like we're dragging our feet.

We do get people shouting at us, 'Come on mate! Get a shift on!' But we're just making sure we're on top of the situation. Or at least appear to be.

I'm trying to talk this lady through what to do when it dawns on me that neither she nor her partner speak English. So I have to act it out instead. I usually don't mind a game of Christmas Day charades, but this is on a different level. I spend about an hour demonstrating heavy breathing and making squeezing faces. It must look like I'm doing my best impression of a turkey, but it seems to be working, so I carry on.

When the baby finally decides it wants to make its entrance, the umbilical cord is wrapped around its neck. We're taught to flick the cord over a baby's head, but I'm not able to. I'm fumbling and starting to panic, but can't let the mum see that. Eventually I manage to get my fingers underneath, reduce the strain and, as a result of one last push, out pops the baby into my arms, like the proverbial bar of soap. Then, silence, which seems to go on for ever.

When you're in hospital and you think there might be something wrong with a baby, you pull a cord and before you know it, every man, woman and their dogs are in the room. But ambulance workers don't have a magic cord. Mercifully, the baby starts crying eventually. I get Dad to cut the cord, dry the baby, wrap him up and pass him to Mum. Mission accomplished.

When a woman has a baby, you can see the change in them immediately. When they look into that baby's eyes for the first time, they forget about everything they've just been through. And so do we. It's just so wonderful to see that instant love and utter devotion. How many people can say when they get home from work, 'I delivered a baby today and brought joy to people's lives'?

I sometimes wonder where that baby is now. I hope he's happy we brought him into the world. But there's no time to stand, stare and wonder when we're wading knee-deep through a twelve-hour shift. There's not even time to return to the station for a brew – those days are gone. The calls are stacked up waiting for us, so that we're almost always on the road, ready to respond. We dispose of our gloves, clean ourselves up and breathe. Two jobs down, on to the next one.

Next up is a 97-year-old lady in a care home who has suffered a stroke. I deal with a lot of strokes. If a patient is treated within four hours of the stroke taking place, the hospital can administer a drug that will hopefully burst the blockage, stop tissue wastage in the brain and restore movement in limbs. If a patient has to wait more than four hours for said treatment, a different treatment will be administered that is less effective. Time is of the essence.

I stagger through the door of the care home with every last bit of kit and caboodle – the day you try to predict what you'll need is the day you leave that all-important piece of equipment in the back of the ambulance. A carer shows us upstairs (people always seem to get ill upstairs) and when we're introduced to the patient, we're relieved to discover that she still has all her faculties. She's lost movement down one side, which is a sure sign of a stroke, but she knows what's going on. The whole time we're assessing her, we're also speaking to her, explaining what we're doing and why we're doing it, to put her at ease. But when we suggest we take her to hospital, she's adamant she doesn't want to go. The mere mention of hospital has turned her to jelly. She's probably thinking, *If they take me there, I might never come out again.*

I completely understand, because that's exactly what can happen. But this lady is within the four-hour treatment window and we want to give her the best possible chance of recovering, so, as far as we're concerned, it's all systems go. If she stays at home, she could die of her symptoms. But if someone doesn't want to go to hospital, we can't take them. We can't force healthcare on people, drag them kicking and screaming into the back of an ambulance (unless a patient doesn't have the mental capacity to make their own decisions, and even then you have to prove it's in their best interests, which makes it a minefield).

Being an ambulance person isn't just tearing about at 100mph, a lot of the time it's about patience and taking the time to explain the benefits of our actions. I spend ten or fifteen minutes addressing the lady's fears, explaining why we should take her in and what they might be able to do to help, and eventually she agrees.

In the back of the ambulance, I can tell she's still anxious. So I decide we need a few tunes. I carry a Bluetooth transmitter that plays music from my phone over the ambulance radio. If we've got kids on board, I might stick on a bit of Peppa Pig. If it's a teenager, I might stick on some hip-hop. If it's an adult, I might stick on some panpipes or whale sounds. Anything that might help to calm them down. In this case, I find some Second World War-era songs on Spotify, press play and the lady goes from being scared out of her wits to singing along to 'We'll Meet Again'. I join in and we end up having the time of our lives. I can't help wondering what she's thinking about while we're singing along to Vera Lynn. Her husband? Old friends long gone? Whatever it is, to turn this horrible experience into a positive one is quite overwhelming.

I love hearing old people's stories from way back when, so I ask the lady what she did during the war. She tells me she worked in a munitions factory, about an explosion that killed a lot of people and how proud she was that she'd played her part. I want to help anyone who ends up in the back of my ambulance, but when it's someone who has given so much, you desperately want to make their experience as comfortable as possible and repay them with your time. Otherwise it can feel like they're part of a factory process, placed on a conveyor belt, quickly checked over, before being rushed back out again.

A few days later, I hear that the lady passed away in hospital, which was her worst fear. But at least I made the end of her journey more bearable, simply by showing how much I cared. That was the best Christmas present I could have given anyone.

As for my presents, I unwrap them while my kids are in bed. I kiss them goodnight, taking care not to wake them, make a turkey sandwich and have a couple of bottles of beer with my wife on the settee. That Christmas Day, I witnessed the start of one life and the end of two others. And whatever the outcome, I tried my very best. It sounds like something worth reflecting on. But reflecting is not something ambulance people do much of. We have private lives to lead, loved ones to look after and Christmas telly to watch.

2

THE HARDEST JOB

I was eighteen years old and thought I knew everything. And then I got a girl pregnant. We weren't really planning a family at that age, so it was kind of unexpected. When I told my mum, I was wearing the same Diadora T-shirt I'd had since I was about thirteen. Mum wasn't exactly over the moon. But she soon calmed down and vowed that we'd bring up the baby between us. Dad is a man of few words. He had even less than usual to say about this particular matter.

My daughter Maddison was a beautiful little thing, an absolute cracker. The one big problem was that me and her mother were just a couple of immature teenagers who didn't get on particularly well. But I thought that I should at least give it a go. I didn't want to be an absent parent and not be part of it, so I thought that maybe we'd spend the first year together, watching our daughter grow up. Then, about eleven months after Maddison was born, my girlfriend became pregnant again. Telling my mum was pretty much the same as the first time, except this time she was even more upset.

A few months later, my girlfriend went for her first scan. The nurse said, 'Right, I can see the baby there.' Before adding, 'Oh, I'll just need to grab a doctor . . .' I was standing there thinking, *What the hell is wrong?* The doctor came in, took one look at the scan and said, 'Congratulations, it's twins.' I went home and said to Mum, 'You know I said she was pregnant again? Well, she still is. But this time there's two of them . . .'

Twenty-seven weeks into the pregnancy, my girlfriend's waters broke and she went into labour. The twins – Rhianna and Courtney – were born thirteen weeks early and transferred straight to intensive care. They looked like little aliens, but they were our little aliens, and we immediately loved them immensely. One of them had a collapsed lung; both of them were on ventilators. The doctor told us they were probably going to die. Never mind how old I was, this type of news would have ripped the heart out of anyone.

I couldn't live at the hospital, or even in my car, because we had another baby to look after. I stayed off work for a bit, but there's only so much leeway your bosses can give you. So after about a month, I had to go back in. I can't blame them. They didn't tell me to have a kid, let alone three in eighteen months.

I was already working for the ambulance service, and had been since two days after my eighteenth birthday, which made me their youngest ever employee. As such, you might think joining the ambulance service was a burning ambition, almost an inevitability. But I stumbled into it.

———

School wasn't really for me. Even at primary school, I struggled to fit in. I remember on a school trip to France, everyone writing down who they wanted to share a room with. The teacher reached the bottom of the list and I was the odd one out. I had a lot of pent-up frustration and would stand my ground. If anyone said anything I didn't like, chances are I'd lump them.

One of my fellow pupil's dads, who was a policeman, took a particular dislike to me. He thought it necessary to visit the headteacher and tell him that, in his professional opinion, I was a bad person, destined to end up in prison and shouldn't be in the school. It's possible I'd punched his son. Mum and Dad were devastated. A copper deciding your son is a wrong 'un carries a lot of weight.

Eventually, I was referred to an educational psychologist and diagnosed with dyslexia. And once that diagnosis was made, the frustration died down. I was given support, which changed everything. Once I understood that there was nothing wrong with me, I started to thrive.

But secondary school wasn't much better. I didn't fit the template of a model student. I struggled to deal with people dictating to me the way things were supposed to be. There were certain things I wasn't willing to accept, so I was always asking why. For example, I hated inequality. From an early age, I thought everybody should be treated the same, regardless of who or how old they were. I didn't understand why we'd all be lining up outside in the rain while the teacher was inside drinking a cup of tea, looking at us through the window. I didn't understand why we weren't allowed to take our blazers off when it was 100 degrees in the classroom. I didn't have an authority problem, I just didn't like being treated differently from adults. A teacher said to me once, 'Stop acting like a child!' I replied, 'Stop treating me like one!' And he replied, 'You'll never be anything in your life if you don't buck up!' I spent the rest of that lesson in the corridor.

So I muddled through school, before leaving with three GCSEs at C or above. I wasn't thick, I just didn't want to be there and couldn't wait to escape. There must be so many kids like me.

My uncle had a plumbing firm, so I started an apprenticeship with him. Summer was great, autumn less so.
Then it got to February. I was carrying some lead up a
ladder, dropped it on my toe and thought, *You know what?*
Sod this. After that day, I never went back. I was already
working weekends at a garden centre to bump up my
wages and now I started working there full-time. I did a
bit of sweeping and hoovering, restocking shelves, helping elderly ladies load compost into their car boots. It was
wonderful, completely stress-free. And zipping around
on the forklift made me feel like a man of the world. The
whole way through secondary school, I'd wanted to be
an adult. And now I was. At least I felt like one. Now I'm
actually an adult, I want to be a kid again.

My next job was working for a travel agency, selling
holidays over the phone. I was trained by some lovely
people, including a guy called Russell, who was an absolute legend and tragically died of an asthma attack some
years later. It was also where I met Neil, who's still my
best mate. I had a whale of a time, but it was commission
based, and I wasn't always available on the phone. I was
busy doing other things, like chasing girls in the café and
enjoying the usual distractions of a teenage boy.

I stayed at the travel agency for a year or so, before
seeing an advert in the newspaper for an emergency medical dispatcher (EMD), answering 999 calls and dispatching

ambulances. I had a bit of telesales experience, quite fancied a job in the services (my parents both worked for the prison service – my mum in HR and my dad taking prisoners out to do community work), so I applied.

Having the opportunity to do something exciting and make a difference appealed to me. This wasn't a case of selling a service to the public; this was a case of the public desperately wanting a service from me. And the pay wasn't based on commission.

Up until this point, though, I hadn't had much to do with the ambulance service, or even the NHS. But when I was working at the garden centre, a sign fell over and hit a lady on the head. What I remember most about that day is that while I was flapping, the person who answered my 999 call was so incredibly calm. That left a lasting impression on me.

I was only seventeen when I went for the interview, so didn't hold high hopes. But the guy who interviewed me recognised my desire and passion and offered me the job. They sent me on a four-week course, where I learned how to answer the calls – 'Pick up the phone. Press that button. Stay calm. Ask these questions, based on the patient's condition. Stay on the line and offer the relevant advice until the ambulance arrives. Put the phone down. And repeat' – and that was pretty much it.

Well, that's not quite true. EMDs are at the lower end

of the ambulance service pay scale, and among its least appreciated employees. When you think of the ambulance service, you don't think of someone sat behind a desk, you think of paramedics bursting through a door, dripping with medical paraphernalia. But being an EMD was the hardest, most stressful job I've ever done. Whereas on the road I might do ten jobs a day, on the phones I might do fifteen jobs in half an hour. And you've got to be achieving. Everything you say can be listened to and a certain percentage of calls are audited, which is why I was a little bit worried the time my tapes got seized by the police for evidence, as they might have heard me ordering prawn crackers, crispy shredded beef, chicken kung po and egg fried rice on the previous call. Well, it was Chinese night. I just hope it never made it to court.

Some of the stuff that happened while I was doing that job was surreal. Someone phoned up and said, 'I know where you're based, I'm gonna be in the car park waiting to kill you when you're finished.' It was often impossible to tell whether my abuser was drunk, high on drugs, had mental health problems or was simply an idiot. People would phone and say, 'Mate, I've got no money for a taxi. You're gonna have to send an ambulance to drop me off at home, otherwise I'm going to die of hypothermia.' What can you say? I couldn't help but despair at times.

Very occasionally, an EMD will take a call that is

horribly close to home. One colleague was on her very first shift when she took a call from her ex-husband, who had taken an overdose. Imagine that. But I also had my own dose of reality. One day, a call came in from my girls' nursery. I asked my colleague for the name of the patient and she said, 'Maddison Farnworth.' My heart sank. I took the headset off my colleague and the caller told me my daughter was having a fit. I legged it out of the office, jumped in the car and slammed my foot down. If a copper had tried to pull me over, he would have had to follow me all the way to the nursery. I wasn't stopping for anyone.

When I got to the nursery, just after the ambulance, I was shaking like a leaf. It turned out my daughter was having something called a febrile convulsion. These happen when a child has a fever and their temperature suddenly rises, sending their body haywire and causing them to have a seizure. They're not usually life-threatening, but I didn't know that, so was absolutely terrified.

I travelled with my daughter in the back of the ambulance, carried her into hospital and when I put her down, the nurse said, 'Leave it with me.'

'No, I'm staying.'

'What do you mean?'

'I'm her dad.'

I forgot I was still in my uniform. The nurse thought I was part of the show.

I delivered a baby over the phone once. I said to the bloke, 'The ambulance is on its way. But it might not make it on time, so I'm going to talk you through it.' That's one of the last things a bloke wants to hear. I told him to grab some towels, and I heard him huffing and puffing up the stairs and rummaging around in his airing cupboard with his phone wedged between his shoulder and his ear. I was sat there thinking, *This is ridiculous. I'm sat here in a bright air-conditioned room drinking a brew and this guy's partner is having a baby.* I could hear screaming and yelping in the background, and eventually a baby crying. Suddenly, that feeling of ridiculousness was replaced by a glow of satisfaction.

One time, a woman called from a motorway hard shoulder. Both her children were unconscious in the back of her car and her husband was drowsy and vomiting. That was a tough job, because it's hard to get a location when someone is on a motorway. Some people don't have a clue where they are and a few don't even know which motorway they're on, which can be very stressful for the EMD and the caller. Having worked out where this lady was, I sent an ambulance out and it transpired that the exhaust was leaking into the car. The kids eventually came to, but if the dad hadn't started vomiting when he did, they might have died, because they looked like they were just sleeping.

Taking those calls was like reading a particularly vivid book. And it was difficult to know whether the pictures I painted in my head were worse than reality or not. I heard some horrific things and had to talk callers through how to administer CPR on numerous occasions. That's a hell of a responsibility, and it comes with a heavy dose of impotence. You can tell people how to do something as clearly and calmly as possible – and you can hear them on the other end of the phone – but you have no idea if they're doing it right.

EMDs hear a lot of screaming and shouting, some of it incomprehensible. But however hysterical the caller was, my job was to stay calm. EMDs are taught 'repetitive persistence' and 'action and reason'. For example, if a caller is screaming down the phone, 'Help, my dad's not breathing!' over and over again, I'd say, 'I need you to give me your address so we can help your dad.' And I'd keep saying it until the caller gave me the information I needed. An EMD's words are fairly scripted, which is why when you listen to 999 documentaries, they often sound quite cold. But if you deviate from the script, you can get into bother. The methods the EMDs use are tried and tested and proven to work, while going off-piste could land you and the patient in trouble.

———

So, this is how I ended up trying to save lives down a telephone, while my twin daughters were fighting for their lives in the hospital. Every now and again someone from the hospital would call to tell us that they'd taken a turn for the worse and we needed to come in immediately. Then they'd rally and I'd go straight back to work. But how are you supposed to concentrate while two of your babies are in intensive care and another one is at home? I was doing twelve-hour shifts, sometimes five days in a row, so I might not see them properly for almost a week. That was soul-destroying.

During that long, agonising period, I became personally acquainted with the NHS and its staff that apparently work miracles, particularly the wonderful doctors and nurses in the neonatal intensive care unit. And eventually, due to their hard work and vigilance, the twins turned the corner. After about six months, they were able to come home, which was an incredible moment. Being able to bring them home was like becoming a father all over again – in more ways than one. Whenever I took them out shopping, I'd have women looking in the pram and saying, 'Oh, look at these beautiful new-born babies!' and I'd have to explain that they were actually born the previous year.

Now I had three babies at home and I was still only twenty. It was very difficult to make sense of it. All I could do was try to keep calm, which was easier said than done. Because just when you think that things can't get any more complicated, life has a habit of chucking a little bit more at you.

3

BURYING TRAUMA

Now me and my girlfriend had three kids together, I thought I needed to make a double effort to keep the relationship going. But things soon started to fall apart, which I had known deep down would happen. It was never going to be easy for a couple so young to bring up three children together. It's not as if somebody up there flicks a switch and turns you into a perfect parent overnight. That takes a great deal of experience. But then there was the time I got stabbed five times by her mystery bloke, which was harder to get my head around.

I'd been working non-stop when one night I decided to go for a meal and a couple of beers with Neil. I had planned to stay at my mum's, but when it got to kicking-out time, I decided I might as well go home and see the kids.

When I arrived at the front door, I could hear my eldest screaming her head off. What on earth was going on here? The front door was locked, and I couldn't get anyone to answer, so eventually I barged it open. I was walking down the hallway when this guy came out of nowhere and attacked me. At first, I thought he'd just punched me, but then I realised I was spurting blood. He'd stabbed me once in the stomach, once in the arm and three times in the chest, before making his escape. Luckily, the last three thrusts of his knife didn't go in. Unluckily, the first two went in quite deep. As I was standing there, I was thinking, *I'm a good guy. I work for the ambulance service. I help people. I don't deserve this.*

I picked up Maddison, gave her a big kiss and a cuddle and said, 'It's okay, darling, he's gone now.' But when I looked down and saw that my white shirt was now red, reality hit. I felt light-headed, nauseous and befuddled. My girlfriend gathered some towels and phoned 999. One of my colleagues took the call, so they knew straightaway it was me.

An ambulance came, whisked me to the hospital and delivered me to the resuscitation room, where doctors administered investigative surgery. While the doctor was digging around in the wounds to find out if any damage had been done to my organs, my control room manager, Tommy, had his hand on my shoulder and made me feel safe. That was a nice touch and something I stored away for later. Thankfully, no major damage had been done. But I still bear the scars to this day, both physical and mental. When the kids ask what happened to me, I tell them I was attacked by a shark.

I didn't phone my mum and dad until about six hours after I'd been stabbed. Mad as it sounds, I didn't want to wake them up in the middle of the night. I'd already put them through the wringer – twice – how were they going to react to this? If you think getting stabbed is bad, try telling your folks. I can laugh about it now. But the reality is, if that knife had gone in much deeper, or centimetres to the left or the right, three little kids would have lost their dad and I wouldn't be telling you this story.

Talk about growing up fast. After I was stabbed, things went a bit jittery, relationship-wise, and I decided it was probably for the best that I end things. I know what some of you older readers are thinking: *These kids give up on relationships too easily nowadays.* But being stabbed can make you see things in a different way. The girlfriend went off and did her own thing, the kids came home with me and I was now a single parent of three children.

My attacker was soon arrested and, two days after being discharged from hospital, I had to traipse down to the police station in absolute agony. I had stitches in my stomach and arm, cuts all over my chest, and every muscle in my body ached. Regardless, this detective gave me the worst grilling I'd ever had: 'Did you approach him first? Did you give him any reason to attack you?' I couldn't believe it. I felt like crying. At the end she said, 'I wasn't doing that to be horrible, but that's what the questioning would be like if the case went to court. Are you prepared for that to happen?' I'd just been stabbed five times and become a single parent to three small children, so I replied, 'You know what, you can stick your court case up your arse, it's not worth the hassle.'

I should have pursued it all the way, and I'll never forgive myself for not doing so. But I just wasn't strong enough, physically or mentally, to fight for justice. As a result, he wasn't charged. His story was that he wasn't aware my girlfriend had a partner and that when he heard someone barging through the door, he grabbed a knife from the kitchen and cut loose. The sad part is, it's entirely plausible. If I'd been in a strange house and heard someone kicking the door in, I might have thought it was an intruder and bashed him over the head with something. I sometimes wonder what he's up to. I only hope he made the most of his second chance.

After the dust had settled, my ex took me to court for full custody. I can only assume that she suddenly had a moment of clarity and realised she'd tossed away a family. Maybe I'm too nice, but I believe that people can change, so I never said she couldn't see her children. But there was no way she was having them full-time. She lost the case, but it wasn't pleasant having it all dredged up again. Family court was a stressful place and not somewhere I ever wanted to return to.

It's difficult to know what kind of psychological effect the attack had on me at the time, because I had no other choice but to bury the trauma. It might sound ridiculous, but other than my family and best mate Neil, I didn't really tell anyone else about it. No one said to me, 'Do you need to speak to someone?' Besides, sharing problems just wasn't my thing, because I didn't think anyone would be interested. I enjoyed listening to other people's stories of glory and woe, and helping out if I could, but I didn't want to burden anyone with mine. Obviously, people knew what had gone on, but when I met my mates down the pub (not that that was a regular occurrence back then anyway, what with having three babies), the extent of the conversation would be, 'You all right? Good. What you drinking?' That's just the way boys deal with things. Or don't.

Me and the kids moved back in with Mum and Dad and they became like a second set of parents. And wonderful parents they were too. They had the loft converted, built an extension out the back and went all out to make everything as comfortable as possible. Most parents will do everything they can for their kids, but what they did was above and beyond the call of duty. I can't even begin to imagine the emotional turmoil I put them through. My sister Lyndsey has a great husband and a perfect family, so I couldn't help thinking that I was a let-down by comparison and an unwanted burden. But they didn't make it about them, they made it about me and their grandchildren. I'd never say everything that happened to me was a good thing, but positives came out of it, including bringing us all closer together as a team.

Unfortunately, my mum was away working at the other end of the country, so the help she could offer with childcare was limited. I managed to get a flexible policy through work, but that didn't go down well with everyone. One female colleague was up in arms that I'd managed to swing a bit of help: 'A bloke with a flexible working policy? Have you ever heard anything so ridiculous? I've been here for thirty years, and I've never had a flexible working policy!' I felt like sitting her down and saying, 'I didn't become a single father of three kids and get stabbed five times on purpose.' But I decided to get my head down and keep plodding. I haven't stopped since.

4

A LIFELONG APPRENTICESHIP

Raising three small children as a young single dad was some of the best training for the frontline of the ambulance service I ever had. My alarm would go off at 6 a.m., I'd roll out of bed, grab the kids, line them up, change their nappies, feed them, get them dressed and stagger to the shower. By the time I'd emerged from the bathroom, they'd all be undressed and one, two or three of them would have done a poo or puked. I'd change their nappies and dress them again, while eating a slice of toast, sling them in the car (not literally, although sometimes I felt like it), drive to the nursery, wait for it to open at eight, hand them over and drive to the other side of town to start work in the control room at 8.30.

At 4.30 p.m., I'd finish my shift, attempt to get to the

nursery before it closed at six, grab the kids, sling them in the car (again, not literally), take them home, feed them, bath them, put them to bed and fall asleep. And the following day, I'd do almost exactly the same all over again. There might be single mothers reading this and thinking, *This is my life!* Well, I tip my hat to you. If you can do that every day without losing your marbles, a career in the ambulance service might be for you.

At the time, I thought that my life had been set in stone, that this would be my existence until the end of days: a grinding cycle of long hours at work and domestic drudgery, which is what bringing up babies often felt like to a kid like me. Of course, it wasn't all a drag. There were those beautiful moments every parent experiences, that made it all seem worthwhile: the first smiles, the first words, the first steps. But it's not like I had much time to savour them.

Luckily, my mum managed to get relocated and started working nearer to home, which eased some of the pressure and even meant I could go for the odd night out with the boys. But it was around this time that I fell ill. My whole body was in pain like you wouldn't believe. Every joint and muscle ached, my knee was swollen up like a balloon and I struggled to get out of bed most mornings.

My doctor referred me to a rheumatologist and he diagnosed something called reactive arthritis, which he said was my body's response to trauma. Apparently – and I had to take his word for it, rheumatology not being my strong suit – my white blood cells, which are there to fight infection, had started attacking my body for the fun of it, because of the stress it had been under. And they'd got so carried away that they'd started having a go at my joints. The rheumatologist put me on immune suppressants, but when I went back to see him, he told me that I needed to return at 9 a.m. the following morning, because if I didn't get my knee drained, I might never walk again.

I was due in work the next day, so I phoned my boss, told him what the rheumatologist had told me, suggested I take the day off as leave, and he told me to stop being so silly: 'It's just a swollen knee. Can't it wait a few days?'

'Not according to the medical professional.'

'Let me have a word with my boss . . .'

About half an hour later, his boss phoned me: 'Dan, John's asked me to call. He's told me he wants you to know that you've got to be in tomorrow. If not, you'll have to face the consequences.'

I can only assume the apparent lack of understanding was down to a breakdown in communications, but I was in so much pain that I couldn't ignore it. So I went sick. And when I next saw my consultant, he signed me off work for six months. I'd had three babies in no time at all, split up with my girlfriend, been stabbed five times and was running around like a blue-arsed fly, trying to care for the kids and bring some money in. I was a complete wreck and agreed with the consultant that I needed a break. Who wouldn't in that situation?

Taking that time off was the best thing I ever did. I was able to have a proper sleep during the day while the kids were at nursery. I was able to spend quality time with them, rather than simply get them dressed, wash them and shovel food down their throats.

Having gone through what I went through, I believe that stress can take a bigger toll on the body than the medical world currently understands, perhaps even kill people. But that break gave me the strength I needed to keep carrying on. The illness slowly dissipated and I became myself again. And feeling refreshed, I applied for a job as an emergency medical technician, on the frontline, because I felt I needed a new challenge to go with a new chapter in my life.

———

To the layman, a technician looks no different to a para-medic. The key differences between a technician and a paramedic are that paramedics receive more training and can administer many more drugs, which are critical in life-threatening situations. But we're both on the frontline together. Technician or paramedic, a lot of people still think of us as ambulance drivers. That's fine with me – we do have to drive the ambulances – but it will upset some of the ambulance service's more sensitive souls. Lots of people also call us first responders, but that's because they watch too much American TV. First responder applies to anyone who is among the first to arrive at an emergency, whether they be a technician, a paramedic, a police officer or a firefighter. (That said, community first responders do exist in the UK, and are volunteers who are dispatched to attend emergencies, often in rural areas, when an ambulance might take longer to arrive.)

When I got the job, I was thrilled. The pay rise was negligible, but I loved the idea of being able to physically help people, rather than blindly guide them over a phone. It takes about ten years to qualify as a GP. If you want to become an anaesthetist, it will take you about fourteen years. Training to be a technician lasts about four months, or at least did in my day. That might not sound very long, but it was very intense, and I had to graft my backside off to pass the course. During those four months, I learned anatomy and physiology; the basic workings of the human body; a manual's worth of medical terminology; how to recognise a host of different illnesses as well as how to treat them; wound care; resuscitation and how to use defibrillators and an ambulance full of equipment; manual moving and handling; infection control and prevention; scene management. Oh, and delivering babies.

Things I didn't learn during training but which might have come in handy included: how to handle being spat at, called every name under the sun, hold a wee for hours at a time, survive hours without an official break and carry patients down spiral staircases. And that's not even the half of it. Real-world incidents are rarely like training scenarios. Perhaps more than any other vocation, being a frontline ambulance clinician is a lifelong apprenticeship – almost every day we are presented with a familiar puzzle assembled in a slightly different way and we have to do what we can to solve it.

The driving course was very full-on, as it should be, given that ambulance folk are allowed to drive with some disregard for the Road Traffic Act. But it was also an enormous amount of fun. We got to drive a skid car, which meant tear-arsing around a disused runway, and the course ended with a time trial. After four weeks, I felt like I could have tackled the Dakar Rally.

When I turned up for my first shift, the paramedic said to me, 'Tell you what, son, you get used to driving this ambulance today and I'll do all the other bits. We'll build it up from there.' But when I jumped in the cab, I said, 'Where's the clutch?' The paramedic chuckled and replied, 'There's no clutch, it's automatic.'

At no point during my training had I driven an automatic ambulance. At no point in my life had I driven any kind of automatic vehicle. I know what you're thinking: the whole point of automatics is that they're a piece of cake to drive. Basically, you rev and go. Unfortunately, where once was the clutch was now a pedal that turned the siren on and off. So every time I thought I was changing gear, the siren started blaring. Thankfully, I understand this slight oversight in our training package has now been reviewed and corrected.

Having informed my partner that, in my hands, the ambulance would perform more like a clown's car, he suggested we grab a brew and take it for a test drive around the station car park. But just as I was getting the hang of things, my first job appeared on the screen: a hot-air balloon had crashed into an electricity pylon and we needed to get there, pronto. My partner said to me, 'You're gonna have to drive with blue lights for this one. I'll talk you through it.' I was thinking, *I didn't see anything about hot-air balloon crashes in the text book*. That said, I couldn't wait to get there and see what was what. Would there be journalists and camera crews? Would it be on the news? This is what I'd envisaged before I'd signed up – helping to save lives at major incidents. I couldn't help thinking of black and white footage from the First World War of burning zeppelins crashing to the ground.

The whole way there, I kept pressing the clutch, which wasn't a clutch but turned the siren on and off: press once and the siren came on, press twice and it played an even more hideous tune, press thrice and it turned off. By the time we arrived at the scene, I thought I'd mastered it. I parked up the ambulance with clammy hands, sweat trickling down my back. I mentally prepared myself for the carnage I might be about to see and ran through the various treatments I might have to administer. It was a case of cometh the hour, cometh the Dan.

I jumped out of the ambulance and made for the back like a greyhound let loose from his trap. Just then a police officer wandered over and said, 'It's all right lads, you're not needed. It came down with a bit of a bump, but nothing serious.' I didn't know if I was relieved, annoyed or frustrated. All the balloon passengers were fine and everyone was calm. That is, until I jumped back into the ambulance, stuck my foot on the 'clutch' and the siren started blaring.

'What the hell are you doing that for?' shouted the copper.

'Because I don't know what the hell I'm doing,' I should have replied. But no one needs to hear an ambulance person say that. So I shrugged instead.

———

Before joining the ambulance service, the only dead body I'd seen was my auntie. She fell down the stairs, was going to die, then wasn't. My mum and dad had arranged to take me and my sister to visit her in intensive care, before getting a phone call to say, 'Leave the kids at home, you need to come and say your goodbyes.' That same day, my auntie passed away. She was thirty-six.

A couple of days later, we visited the funeral home. Mum and Dad gave me and my sister the choice of whether we wanted to see our auntie or not, and I decided to take a look and say goodbye. She'd been cleaned up by the undertaker and given a bit of make-up, but when I looked at her, I froze. She was still someone I knew, but it wasn't her any more. It was a bit late for goodbyes. To be honest, it creeped me out. I had nightmares for weeks.

Seeing my first dead body on the job is etched on my mind. I'm in the station – back in the days when we spent time in the station – the radio starts crackling, and me and my partner, an experienced paramedic, calmly make our way to our ambulance and hop in. I say 'calmly', but my legs feel like fag ash. And when I see the job on the dispatch screen – MALE, CARDIAC ARREST – it feels like my head might explode. Before you do your first job of the day, you are required to log in using a pin number. I've forgotten mine. So there I am, fumbling through my diary, trying to find it. I desperately need the toilet. I believe this is what is technically known as 'shitting oneself'.

It's a short drive to the job with blues and twos (lights flashing and sirens blaring). When we arrive on the scene, my partner jumps out of the ambulance and heads for the front door of the house, while I follow with all the equipment clanging against my hips and knees. The patient's wife is waiting for us in the living room. She matter-of-factly informs us that her husband is upstairs in the bedroom, so my partner asks her to lead the way. As soon as my partner sees the lady's husband, laid on the bed, he knows he's already dead. I thought people died with their eyes shut, but this guy is staring straight at the ceiling. As gently as I can, I ask the lady to return downstairs so that we can assess her husband.

My partner asks if I've seen a dead body before. I tell him I haven't, apart from my auntie, and she was in a coffin. It doesn't look like a person. It's just the shell of someone who had been using that body and recently checked out. I'm wearing rubber gloves, but I'm scared to touch it. My partner, sensing my discomfort, calmly talks me through the symptoms of death, including how to check for rigor mortis. Before then, I thought rigor mortis made a body shake. I must have seen a film or something in which a corpse was twitching. But rigor mortis just stiffens the joints, hence the phrase, 'stiff as a board'.

I'm stood there like a lemon thinking, *What happens next?*, when my partner does something that's humbling: he closes the man's eyes, to make it look like he's doing nothing more dramatic than having a nice snooze. As he's doing it, he chats to the body: 'I'm just gonna shut your eyes, me old mate, to make you look a bit more peaceful . . .' That little act of making the man look like he's asleep instead of dead might save his family some anguish. Yes, he's gone, but at least they can say he went in his sleep. My partner is treating this man with so much respect, almost like he's still alive. To the extent that I'm thinking, *Is he?* I suppose that's the point: dead or alive, he's still a person.

Back downstairs in the living room, my partner breaks the bad news to the dead man's wife: 'Unfortunately, your husband has passed away in his sleep. We don't know what happened, but it was sudden and peaceful, and he wouldn't have known anything about it.' He's just so caring and his actions teach me a valuable lesson that I will never forget: an ambulance person's job isn't just to treat the injured and sick, or deal sensitively with the dead, it is also to bring calm and dignity and counsel the bereaved. I learn more in those few minutes than in the whole of my four or five months of training.

5

An Alarming Regularity

It's impossible to mentally prepare yourself for what you might see as an ambulance worker. Some might argue that's a good thing. If someone said to you, 'In five hours, you'll be sent to a five-year-old boy who's not breathing,' chances are that by the time you turned up, you'd be a nervous wreck.

Ever since switching to the frontline, I'd been worried about how I might react to having to deal with a stabbing, given what had happened to me. But when the inevitable call came in, there was no time to be nervous or upset. The adrenalin was pumping, because I knew I'd have to be in tip-top form. But I also slipped straight into work mode, completely focused on the job in hand.

A lad has been stabbed behind the bins at the bottom

of some high-rise flats. When we arrive on the scene, he's slumped over and full of holes, like a cheese grater. He must be about nineteen, the same age as me when I got attacked. But I don't have the luxury of reflection, because this kid's life is in our hands.

A stabbing is one of the jobs where an ambulance person can make a big difference. The decisions we make in the first couple of minutes after arriving on the scene – about which wound to pack first, which drugs to administer and in what dosages – will potentially save the patient's life. Or not. Although sometimes we can't do anything to help – for example, if the aorta, the largest artery which runs straight down the middle of the body, is severed.

My partner and I do everything we can. We can't really diagnose the big stuff, such as whether his organs are damaged. The doctors and specialists at the hospital will discover the real extent of the trauma. What we need to do is stop this kid from bleeding out on to the floor and dying at the scene. We pack the wound with dressing, including haemostatic gauze, which coagulates the blood. We also administer a drug that helps stem the bleeding. Thankfully, it doesn't appear that his lungs have been damaged, because that would mean sticking a needle in his chest and letting the air out, which is not a nice thing to do – especially on someone still conscious. The whole time we're talking to him, telling him loudly and clearly to stick with us, because while all his other senses might have left him, he can still hear. After giving him some fluids, we put him in the ambulance and hot-foot it to hospital. It isn't until afterwards that I think, *Shit, that kid was me not so long ago*. I can literally feel his pain. Thankfully, and also like me, he lives to fight another day.

———

Gallows humour, however dark and seemingly callous or inappropriate, is as essential to an ambulance person as body armour is to a soldier or a shield is to a riot police officer. Gallows humour is one of the few coping strategies we have, and acts as a buffer between us and the reality of what we're dealing with. So, for example, if we're sent to a bloke who's drunk and on the deck, we might refer to it as a 'PFO' – Pissed and Fallen Over. And if we're sent to an elderly lady who's taken a tumble, we might refer to it as a 'Granny Down'.

Now, before anyone starts penning a letter of complaint to my publisher, I should at this point say that I love grannies to bits. They're always grateful to see us and once we've got them up and put them back in their chair (assuming they haven't done themselves a mischief), we often stick around, make them a cup of tea and natter about old times. Although, I'm not going to lie to you, I don't have the same affection for the PFO.

The ambulance service isn't like *Inspector Morse* or *The Sweeney*, where the characters work with the same partner all the time. That could never happen, simply because people work different shift patterns. But there are colleagues you pair up with more often than others. One of my regular partners was Paul, who ended up being a great pal in and out of work. We used to go for breakfast together and he'd tell me about his life, which was apparently quite turbulent. He always called me 'brother' in his text messages and we became close enough that I suppose you could call our relationship a bromance.

Paul had a particularly wicked sense of humour. Before he joined the ambulance service, he worked as a lifeguard at a swimming pool. One day, he and his mate dressed up a CPR mannequin, tied a rope around its neck and hung it from the ceiling. Obviously, when their other colleague discovered it, he almost keeled over with fright. But when Paul and his mate heard the commotion and wandered in, they pretended they couldn't see anything: 'What are you on about? There's nobody there . . .' That's what you call a dark sense of humour and probably why he fitted right in when he joined the ambulance service.

Paul could be a bit of a nightmare to work with, mainly because I found him so funny. He could also get a bit giddy at times. One night, he was so keen to finish on time that he attempted a sharp turn and got the front of his ambulance stuck on someone's front lawn. Eventually, the whole vehicle was on there, from where he'd tried to nudge it forwards and backwards. Paul was there for about two hours before the recovery man arrived to tow him out.

Whoever I'm working with, I might start giggling at the most inappropriate times. We might be working on a patient, chatting about what went on at the works do and some piece of scandal will crease us up. Very occasionally, something inappropriate will slip out. One time, we turned up to a lady in a fortune-telling booth. While I was checking her over, I couldn't resist saying, 'If you can see into the future, why weren't you already at the hospital when you started getting chest pains?' I said it with a smile and she found it funny. But maybe I shouldn't have said it at all.

But, at least as far as I'm concerned, an ambulance person has to grab every bit of light relief they can, because those nice little chats with grannies are all too rare and those little pockets of humour are like pretty bubbles floating in the air – there one second, gone the next, replaced by a deafening clap of thunder. Laughter is the mind's antiseptic cream and gallows humour is our coping mechanism, no different to soldiers trying to take their minds off the realities of their job with sick pranks and dark jokes.

It's a run-of-the-mill day. You know the drill by now. Me and my partner have just got an elderly lady back to her feet, brushed her off, called her neighbours and made them all a brew, when a shout comes up on our screen with a pub's address. We turn on the hooters and tooters, head for the pub and the details appear: FEMALE COVERED IN BRUISES AND BLOOD. I'm with a paramedic I've never worked with before, but that doesn't matter. Like soldiers in a crack unit, we mix and match, because we have an almost telepathic understanding and instinctively know what each other is capable of.

We both know something is badly amiss before we arrive on the scene, simply from the job description. Anyone covered in bruises and blood is never a good thing. We pull up outside the pub, an ambulance car paramedic waves us in and we grab our gear and follow him upstairs. In a utility room off the corridor, a woman has been beaten to death. Sometimes, the job descriptions that appear on our screens are a little bit understated, and we can immediately tell she's been dead for some time. But she still looks scared. She'd been found by her son, who was asleep in his bedroom when the murder took place. The family dog was in there with her. As we're appraising the scene, the woman's other son turns up with his girlfriend. I intercept them at the top of the stairs and lead them to the furthest room from the murder scene. As we all sit down on the sofa, I still haven't worked out how I'm going to break the news to them.

How are you supposed to tell someone something like that? I have no idea, because I haven't been taught. Frontline ambulance staff still aren't taught today. That's remarkable, given that it's the worst thing someone will ever hear. Not only that, but the way someone is dealt with in the first few hours after receiving terrible news can have a big impact on how they heal. Today, I take a lot of pride in having a caring manner, but I had to stumble across my own technique, having consciously and unconsciously picked up skills from more experienced colleagues. In this particular case, I take a deep breath and just go for it: 'I'm really sorry, but unfortunately your mum has passed away. It would appear she was the victim of an assault.' I think – I hope – I do okay.

The son is obviously very upset but manages to hold it together. He tells us that his mum's boyfriend had a habit of knocking her about and that it was no doubt him who killed her. As he's telling us this, he picks up a cushion and places it on his knee. Underneath where it had been is a large blood stain. Thankfully, and inexplicably, neither the son or his girlfriend notice, and I'm able to discreetly cover the stain with another cushion. Presumably, the woman was murdered on the sofa before being dragged into the utility room. And it suddenly dawns on me that we're sitting slap-bang in the middle of a crime scene and potentially destroying vital evidence.

If we can save someone, the fact that it's a crime scene goes out of the window. But in this case, I immediately realise I've made a category one balls-up. I can feel my trousers getting wet with what I assume is blood. And when the police arrive, I shuffle out of the room backwards. I quietly explain to a copper what has happened, and to say he isn't happy doesn't even begin to cover it. He obviously can't give me a bollocking there and then, but his eyes are ablaze and his features twisted into a look of utter contempt. The copper asks the son and his girlfriend to go downstairs before informing his sergeant that two idiot ambulancemen have done their best to contaminate the crime scene.

The copper soon returns to give me a load of grief and tells us we should have left the building immediately after discovering the body. This is all well and good but leaving the building would have meant exposing the murdered woman's son and his girlfriend to all the rubberneckers gathered outside.

As we're waiting for the copper's sergeant to get back to him, we hear on his radio that someone has phoned the police control room and admitted to murdering someone. I naively think that that will be that, but the sergeant radios in to relay the order that the idiot ambulancemen will have to remove their clothes, so that they can be submitted as evidence.

'He wants us to take our uniforms off?' I ask the copper.

'Yes, like he said, take them off.'

'So you want me to drive back to the station in my pants?'

'I'll see if I can find you something to wear . . .'

A few minutes later, another copper appears carrying an evidence bag and a couple of Tyvek suits (those white zip-up coveralls you've seen on *CSI*). When I take my trousers off, I discover my pants are also soaked in blood, which is every bit as unpleasant as it sounds. At least they haven't got holes in. When we emerge from the pub in our Tyveks and climb into the ambulance, bystanders are looking at us in bemusement, as if to say, 'What the hell has gone on in there? And what have they done with the ambulancemen?'

Because the boyfriend confesses, we don't end up giving evidence in court. But this is one story I'm able to follow to its conclusion via the newspapers. The victim and her boyfriend were planning to open the pub together, up until the night the murder took place. They apparently had a row, she revealed she'd been unfaithful, he flipped and stabbed her multiple times in the neck and eye, before strangling her. That's the sight that greeted us. About half an hour before the attack, she had woken her son, given him a hug and told him she loved him. She was forty-four.

The one piece of good news, if you can call it that, was that her killer got charged with murder and banged up for life.

———

These 999 documentaries you see on TV don't really tell the full story, at least not as far as the ambulance service is concerned. They do give an insight into the stresses of the job, but their framing is very narrow. I appeared in the first series of the Channel 4 show *999: What's Your Emergency?* and they usually only showed one of my jobs a week. And it was always a varnished version of what took place. For example, when they filmed us doing CPR, they wisely chose not to broadcast the patient's face, with their eyes wide open and staring straight into mine. They didn't film a dead baby or someone who had been catapulted through a car windscreen. I understood why, because it would have been unethical, and nobody in their right mind would have wanted to watch it. Nevertheless, it would have been a more honest portrayal, because that's the sort of thing ambulance people see with alarming regularity.

One night, the documentary makers are desperate to get footage of the police, fire and ambulance services setting off from their respective bases and arriving at the scene of an emergency together. A camera crew has been out with us all night but decides to give up the ghost and knock off ten minutes early. Big mistake. A few minutes later, a call comes in for a house fire, which is why, unlike telly people, we don't have the luxury of cutting a shift short.

Normally when a call comes in for a house fire, it goes straight to the fire service, they deploy and pass the job on to us. But on this occasion, for reasons unknown, we get the call first. The first thing I want to see when I turn up to a house fire is a fire engine, because ambulances don't have hose pipes. What are we going to do, chuck a glass of water on it? But when we pull into the street, we can see fire and lots of smoke – but no engine. My heart falls into my stomach. My stomach struggles to digest it.

It's seven in the morning, but the whole street is out. People are crying, wringing their hands and running around in panic. The fact that people are shouting 'Help him! Help him!' tells us that someone is probably inside. People see us in our uniforms and automatically think that we can help in any situation. But if someone has a heart attack on a plane, no one will ask if there is a traffic warden on board, on the basis that they wear a uniform as well.

I look at the burning house, thinking, *What the hell am I gonna do here? I've got to do something. I can't just stand here like a lemon.* I snap some rubber gloves on, walk up to the door, touch the handle and my glove gets stuck. While I'm trying to pull my glove off, I can see the silhouette of a figure through the glass pane. Me and my partner discuss kicking the door in, but because we've both seen the film *Backdraft*, we decide that if we do kick the door in, we might get sucked in or incinerated by escaping flames. I'm also thinking, *I don't want to die, I've got three kids at home.*

I'm about to be consumed by my impotency when Trumpton, as we call the fire service, appear on the scene (both the ambulance service and police refer to our friends in the fire service as this, after the old kids' TV programme, or the water fairies, largely out of jealousy). I breathe a huge sigh of relief. A couple of firefighters jump out of the engine, smash a window and neither of them gets sucked in or incinerated. A few seconds later, the firefighters reappear, carrying a smouldering body. In the poor person's outstretched hand is a set of keys. He'd obviously been trying to get to the door when he was overcome and was only a few feet from making it.

Having made certain the poor man is dead and there is nothing we can do to help, we clock off for the day and return to our respective homes. When I wake a few hours later, I switch on my phone and have about thirty missed calls, twenty voicemails and umpteen text messages. What the hell's gone on? A terrorist attack? A multi-vehicle pile-up? None of that. I'm in the latest copy of *Heat* magazine, sitting pretty at the top of their 'Manometer', just above Gok Wan. Every cloud and all that.

I roll out of bed, chuck on some clothes, pick the kids up

from school and put on my smiley face. If anyone asks how work has been, I reply: 'Fine.' What else am I supposed to say? 'Bloody brilliant. This guy died in a house fire. He was smoking when they dragged him out, with his door key in his hand ...' That sort of chat can be difficult to digest with your roast dinner.

6

FACES QUICKLY FADE

In fairness to the system, there is no amount of training that will prepare you for a job on the frontline of the ambulance service. It's sink or swim, and if you don't learn fast, you will plummet to the bottom, maybe while clutching a P45.

While most bodies work – or don't – in the same way, every personality is different. As such, 99 per cent of the job is talking to people in the right way, what you might call the softer skills. We're trained to recognise heart attacks, treat strokes and dress wounds, but that person who comes off his bike and snaps his femur, or trips, falls through a window and cuts herself, needs comforting as well as patching up.

We also find ourselves dealing with deeper societal issues – relationship problems, domestic violence, drug and alcohol addictions and, on occasion, someone who has announced they're feeling suicidal on Facebook or Twitter. As such, ambulance people have no choice but to be everything from medical professionals to social workers to vicars to crowd control.

What I've learned is that if you treat every patient as if they were a member of your own family, you can't go far wrong. How many times have you heard a friend or relative say, 'The ambulance people were just so lovely'? Hopefully, you've heard it a lot. If that's one of a patient's main takeaways from one of our visits, then we've done our job properly. If not, we haven't.

Some of what we do can be quite invasive, especially as a male dealing with a female patient. In those situations, it's about being respectful and clear, explaining exactly what we're doing and why we're doing it. If a patient is having a suspected heart attack, I'll do an ECG (electrocardiogram), which involves attaching little pads around the left side of the chest. But I don't just whip a patient's top up and start slapping these pads on. That's unlikely to go down too well. Instead, I'll explain why they'll benefit from an ECG, because it will give us an indication of what's going on with their heart. Then I'll tell them what an ECG involves, before employing some distraction techniques, trying to make a patient think that what I'm doing is as humdrum as buttoning up a shirt, just general chit-chat, like asking what's cooking in the kitchen or where they bought their stereo.

Sometimes, I receive letters from mums and dads, thanking me for being so good with their children, which is gratifying. You can't treat kids the same as you treat adults. I once saw a programme where they dressed a kid up in an astronaut suit before putting him through an MRI scanner, which they told him was a spaceship. Suddenly, a serious procedure was a bit of fun. I love stuff like that. An emergency can be terrifying for a kid. All they want is their mummy or daddy, and suddenly two strange people in uniforms walk through the door, carrying a load of weird kit. So we have to become something like entertainers (don't worry, I never go full David Brent: 'I'm a friend first and an ambulance person second. Probably an entertainer third . . .'). When we deal with kids, we often deal with hysterical parents, or at least parents who are struggling to hold things together. I understand that it can be traumatic seeing your child in distress. But if you keep a kid calm, usually their parents will stay calm as well.

Treating children can be very rewarding. It's all about doing whatever you can to make it feel like a game. While I'm assessing them, I might ask who their favourite cartoon character or footballer is. I might give them an instrument to play with and have a bit of banter:

'You need to hold this red light for me ... actually, I'll give it to Mum ...'

'No! I want it!'

'All right. But first, I bet you can't sit still while I put it in your ear ...'

Sometimes, I'll give a kid my phone to play with. It's amazing what kids will do for a bit of YouTube. *Calamity Crow* is one of my favourites. It's a cartoon about a crow. Who has calamities. It's brilliant.

I'll say to the kid, 'You remind me of someone I know.'

'Who?'

'Calamity Crow.'

'Who's he?'

'You've never heard of Calamity Crow? Have a look at this ...'

And I'll give them my phone, stick on *Calamity Crow* and get cracking with what we need to do. I might be dressing a wound, and the kid will be singing along with the theme tune. Tactics, that's what it is.

It could be argued that you can't teach anyone how to break bad news, because there are just so many different possible scenarios. If we turn up and someone is already dead, we might simply say, 'Unfortunately, your husband has passed away.' If we turn up, attempt to save them and can't, we might say, 'We've done everything we can, but his heart has stopped. We could continue, but it's very unlikely his heart will restart.' But the words aren't set in stone and are only part of the equation.

What you say to a 90-year-old lady whose husband has just died, and how you say it, is often very different to what you say to a 30-year-old woman whose child has just died. The former is more likely to be calm and resigned, the latter to be hysterical and disbelieving. Working for the ambulance service, you become extremely versatile. We work things out as we go along and hope that we can adapt to any eventuality.

———

Trundling along one fine afternoon, a strange call comes in: MAN FOUND FACE DOWN IN PUDDLE, CARDIAC ARREST. That's all we have. We're about twenty minutes away, so I deliver a heavy right foot and get the ambulance moving. If someone is face down in a puddle, we want to get there as soon as possible. We only hope the caller has pulled him out. We don't want someone drowning in a puddle on our watch.

The satnavs in ambulances are programmed automatically, which is wonderful: when a job comes in, we don't have to muck about entering postcodes and addresses, we can just get on our way. However, the satnavs have a strange glitch, whereby they take you to the middle of properties, which sometimes means you end up being directed down a little alley that runs past the back door, rather than the whacking great, ambulance-friendly road that runs past the front. It happens enough that we have a name for it: the back-door boogie. On this occasion, the poor ambulance doesn't have a choice, because it turns out the poor chap is face down in a puddle on a bridle path.

How do you get a 5-ton ambulance down a bridle path? That's not the start of a joke. The answer is you try to avoid smashing into every overhanging branch and bouncing in and out of every pothole, while hoping you don't end up in a ditch full of mud and all your equipment is in one piece when you arrive at the scene. After some tense exchanges between me and my partner, centred on the belief that we might be on the wrong bridle path, perhaps in the wrong town, we see a woman with a dog frantically waving at us in the distance. We're in the right place, which is always handy when you're desperate to save someone's life.

The woman leads us to the man, who is still face down in a puddle. To be fair, it's quite a big puddle, about 15ft wide and 6 inches deep. We wade out, roll the patient halfway over and it's immediately obvious that not only is he not moving, he's dead. The two things are probably related. He has a head injury, so I assume he's tripped, knocked himself out, landed face down in the puddle and drowned. We all hope to die peacefully at home in our sleep, sat in our favourite armchair in front of a roaring fire, a rug over our knees and surrounded by beaming relatives. Sadly, not many people go out in such a dignified fashion. Still, this is a particularly unlucky way to make an exit.

The guy has white hair, is well dressed and floating next to him is a gold-topped walking cane. He must have been there for a while, because rigor mortis has set in. Because it's an unexpected death, it's now a crime scene. That means we have to leave him as he is, face down in the puddle, so that the police can attend, arrange for crime scene investigation (CSI) to do their thing and hopefully rule out foul play.

While waiting for the police to arrive, we do our best to block off the path, using our vehicle and an ambulance car that is also on the scene. But that doesn't stop people trying to get through. It never does. Most people get it. You say to them, 'The path is currently closed due to an incident,' and they give you a knowing nod and find an alternative route. Other people are less compliant. The conversation will go something like this:

'Sorry, you don't want to go down there, there's been an incident.'

'I'm trying to walk my dog here, mate. This is all I need.'

'Not today, sir. Can you find another way?'

'No. I go this way every day.'

And with that, they'll barge past you. I might feel like saying, 'Listen, pal, there's a man down there dead in a puddle. If your kids see him, they'll have nightmares for weeks. Stop being an idiot and go another way.' But I can't say that, because I'd probably end up in a spot of bother. And we have no real power to stop the public doing what they want to do anyway.

While we're trying to manage the scene, a Toyota Yaris pulls up, an elderly lady climbs out and says, 'I'm looking for my husband. He's got dementia and has gone missing. I got in the shower and when I got out, he'd gone.' I ask what her husband looks like and she says, 'He's got white hair and walks everywhere with a gold-topped cane.'

The obvious thing to say is, 'Oh, he's just over there, in a puddle.' Which is true. A tempting thing to say is, 'I haven't seen anybody with white hair and a gold-topped cane.' Instead, I tell her we're dealing with a man who has been found deceased, and she instantly understands that it's probably her husband. Still, I decided it's better to break the terrible news in a more ideal setting.

I sit her in the passenger seat of her car and drive us back to her house. If I have a prang, I'll probably end up in hot water, but I can't have her behind the wheel. She keeps firing questions at me and I keep stonewalling. As soon as I walk in the house, I see a picture of the woman and a man who is presumably her husband. They are on a cruise together, with big smiles on their faces. I can categorically say that the man in the picture is the man we've found.

While I'm making the lady a cup of tea, I phone my partner: 'It's definitely him. What should I do?'

The police still haven't turned up, so I sit the woman down, take a deep breath and say, 'We can't say for sure, but I'm confident the man we found is your husband.' By now, I've worked with a lot of fine paramedics, watched and learned and polished my technique. I speak softly, take it slowly, explain clearly what has happened and give it time to sink in. I leave out the part about finding him in a puddle.

The woman starts sobbing and I put a consoling arm around her. She is so upset that she had that shower and left him unsupervised. She'll probably carry that guilt for as long as she lives. When she's calmed down a bit, she gives me her daughter's phone number. I give her a call, explain the circumstances and she says she's on her way. Unfortunately, she lives about five hours away. I ask the lady if she has any friends nearby, and she says there might be one at the bowling club around the corner. So I get on my toes and head for the bowling club.

When I walk through the door, all these women start panicking. I imagine when you reach a certain age, an approaching ambulance person with their head bowed and wearing a serious face looks a lot like the Grim Reaper, come to bring tidings of a dead partner or friend. Mercifully, I've left my scythe in the ambulance. I identify the friend I'm looking for, tell her what has happened and walk her back to the lady's house. The whole way there I'm thinking, *I really hope it was her husband, otherwise I'll have some explaining to do.*

While we're waiting for the police to arrive, it suddenly occurs to me that I've been in this house before. A few years earlier, I treated a gentleman with chest pains. He didn't have dementia then. The woman's friend explains that he had a sudden onset and was on a waiting list to see a social worker. I leave with the parting words, 'Sorry to meet you in such sad circumstances, take care.' I shudder to think how many times I've uttered that sentence in the past fifteen years.

When I get back to the body, a CSI photographer is snapping away. Once enough pictures have been taken, the decision is made to put the chap in the ambulance and transfer him to a mortuary. It's never a job I relish. Whenever we've got a dead body on board, I always feel like one of us should sit back there and keep them company. Mad as it might sound, it just seems like the right thing to do.

It's quite rare that I have to go to the mortuary thank God. A mortuary is such a sad place. Rows of dead heads and dead feet and a separate fridge labelled: 'Children Only'. Most people today, at least in the developed world, are so removed from death. It's not the norm any more, as it was for previous generations, to see dead bodies, to the extent that it's quite possible to live a whole life without seeing one. But a trip to the mortuary hammers home just how commonplace death is. I reckon most people working on the frontline of the ambulance service would have had the thought at least once: *I should have gone into the funeral game, I would have made a fortune.*

We unload our body, the mortuary workers place it on a slab and slide it into a chamber. We sign the necessary forms, say our goodbyes and it's only when I get back in the ambulance that it hits me how cruel life can be. It was heart-breaking to be there when that long and loving marriage came to a juddering halt. I pop into people's lives and might only be there for a few minutes before popping off again. But in that short flash of time, I bear witness to monumentally important moments and leave an enduring mark, which is a very humbling thought. Most of the time we can make a positive differ-ence, though sometimes nature beats us to it. But even if it does, those few minutes following an accident, or a tragedy, can still make the rest of someone's life more bearable. That's why what we do is so much more than just a job.

———

The day after the man in the puddle, I took my little boy to the toy shop. In the car park, a woman came up to me and said, 'Oh, hello. How are you?' I must have looked blank, because she followed up with the classic, 'You don't remember me, do you?' She explained that I'd visited her mum a few times and, as you do, I pretended that I suddenly remembered who she was talking about.

'Oh, yes! How is she?'

'She passed away last year.'

'Oh, that's a shame. She was such a lovely lady.'

You say what you've got to say, because doing anything different will make you look callous or uninterested. But I'd be lying if I said that all of the people I treat become more than individual jobs. I'll be in the supermarket doing my big shop and someone will come up to me and say, 'Bloody hell, you're the fella who helped me out the other week!' And I'll look at them and think, *Nope, I have absolutely no idea who you are.*

I deal with so many different people in so many different situations and, to a certain degree, most humans look the same. I remember houses – a fish tank in a living room, a picture in a hallway, a car parked in the driveway – but faces quickly fade. Not remembering makes me feel guilty. But I just have to tell myself that it's no different to being a teacher: some kids they remember years later, some kids they don't. It doesn't make sense to feel guilty, as long as I did everything I could to help.

7

MAKING ME DESPAIR

An ambulance person doesn't always know what they're getting themselves into. A job appears on the screen, say for example: MALE COLLAPSED ON THE STREET. But there are lots of different reasons men collapse on the street. It could be for a variety of medical reasons, or because they've drunk far too many shots. Or they might have been punched unconscious. Or maybe they've tripped and hit their head on the kerb. Another call might say: FEMALE FALLEN OVER IN HOUSE. And when we get there, she's clearly been assaulted. We'll sit her down and ask whether she wants to talk about or report what actually happened. But we can't make them.

We might get called to someone who has reported a chest pain and when we turn up, they've got a knife sticking out of their chest. Or we'll be called to someone who can't get out of bed, and when we arrive, they'll be a bariatric patient (the medical term for morbidly obese). You can almost guarantee that their flat will be on the top floor and the lift won't be working.

When I started out in the job, we weren't provided with any specialist equipment to deal with this, partly because obesity wasn't as big a problem, partly because society was simply less understanding. So the first bariatric job I went to, I walked into this woman's bedroom, saw her on the bed and thought, *How the hell are we gonna get her out?* She must have been 30 stone, at least, so wasn't able to get up, let alone get down the stairs. But we knew we had to get her to hospital for a blood test pronto, because she was complaining of chest pains. We also knew that our only option was to call the fire service, because we didn't have the necessary kit.

Despite the difficulties I could see were going to be involved in getting the patient out, we did everything we could to make her feel at ease. Every time a clinician meets a patient, they should introduce themselves. It sounds like a no-brainer, but in the fog of a day's work, people forget themselves. The patient in question no doubt felt vulnerable and exposed, lying on her bed with nothing but a sheet to protect her modesty. But me saying, 'Hi, my name's Dan and this is my colleague

Paul,' hopefully made the situation feel a little bit less intimidating for her. And when the fire brigade turned up, we introduced them to the patient one by one. Being on first name terms removes barriers and makes everyone involved feel more comfortable.

Once we'd broken the ice, I explained to the lady why we needed to take her to hospital and that it was going to be a bit tricky to get her out of the house and into the ambulance. I think I said something along the lines of, 'It's going to take some working out, so you'll have to bear with us. But I'm sure we'll be able to get you to where you need to be safely.' You have to be honest, but you can sugar the pill by saying it gently.

We tried to make sure we had our plan worked out beforehand, because we didn't want to be having urgent conversations while we were standing over her, scratching our heads, huffing and puffing and generally making it sound like a major operation. That's likely to make a patient feel like they're putting us out.

As always, we involved the patient in our discussions: 'What if we do this? Would it be okay if we did that?' Otherwise, she'd feel like a spare part, as if we're moving an inanimate object. The key thing to remember in any situation like this is that we're dealing with a real person, not a piano, and it's important that they feel a part of their own treatment, rather than a nuisance.

However, the fire service had to use what appeared to be a horse net to lift her off the bed, because they weren't provided with the necessary equipment either. It took about ten firefighters to carry her out and down the stairs. We removed the stretcher from the back of the ambulance and they replaced it with her mattress, so that she had something to lie on. The fire engine followed us to the hospital, used the net to remove her from the ambulance and I can't even remember how they got her inside. Some things are best forgotten.

Whatever your views on obese people – and I realise some people don't have much sympathy for them – that's no way to treat anyone. It wasn't our fault, and it wasn't the firefighters'. None of us had the tools. But every patient should be treated with respect and dignity. And putting someone in a net is not treating them with the respect or dignity they deserve.

Thankfully, things have changed significantly. Now, there are special bariatric ambulances and chairs with caterpillar tracks that carry the patient up and down stairs. We call it the 'electric chair', although not within earshot of the patient. That would be one way to finish someone off with a heart attack. Most of the time now we can do the job without having to call the fire service, but the electric chair will only work on wide staircases with not too many turns. If that's the case, the fire service will get the patient out using a specialist slide sheet, which is a bit more dignified than a net.

But you still hear stories about doors, windows and even walls having to be removed in order to extract a bariatric patient from their house. Some of these extractions are logistical nightmares and can take more than a day, because sometimes supporting systems will have to be put in the house to ensure that everything stays structurally sound and the whole thing doesn't come crashing down. And you can bet your life the fire service doesn't put it all back together again when you get out of hospital. You'll have to get a builder in for that, and they cost money.

Obviously, the main causes of obesity are lack of exercise and overeating. But why is someone not exercising and overeating to such an extent? It's often a result of medical or mental health problems rather than pure greed. The bigger they get, the less confident they become, so they become prisoners in their own homes. And because of the internet, they don't have to go out to the shops or leave the house to socialise, so it's a vicious circle. It's a crying shame that the root causes of their obesity aren't spotted earlier. How can society allow it to reach the point where someone can't get out of bed?

Ideally, there would be more work in communities, people teaching preventive measures, the perils of a bad diet, smoking, too much booze and lack of exercise. It would certainly make our job easier on the body (when we're faced with bariatric patients, we don't hang around doing limbering-up exercises, like weightlifters, we have to get straight to it) and it would save the NHS an awful lot of money.

While some people eat themselves to death, others prefer drink. Ambulance people see every stage of an alcoholic's decline, from their early days on the bottle, when they're falling unconscious and needing reviving, to when they've turned yellow because their liver is starting to fail, to when they're vomiting blood because of oesophageal varices, which basically means the veins in their oesophagus have ruptured. That's one of the worst things an ambulance person can see. Me and Paul were on a job once and we turned up to find the patient's living room looking like a scene from *The Exorcist*. There was blood everywhere and I could see the abject fear in his eyes, because oesophageal varices can hit you from nowhere. But there was nothing we could do, other than get him in the ambulance and go.

I get to see how people from every sector of society live. Some people live in luxury. The vast majority have comfortable, clean, tidy homes. People at the bottom live in total squalor. I'll walk into a house and there will be mould on the ceiling, floorboards missing, windows boarded up and doors hanging off hinges. And at least one of those doors usually has a fist-sized hole in it.

How some people live is nothing short of tragic. I was

called out to one house and when the copper answered the door, he was kneeling on top of a pile of rubbish that must have been 4ft high. We climbed on top and crawled after this police officer, as if we were potholing. We didn't know what we were crawling over. There could have been needles sticking out, animal excrement and rats sniffing about. We found the elderly lady in what we think was her bedroom, already dead. But what I remember most about that job was the fact we could hear the TV but not see it. That TV must have been on for years, because there was no way she could have switched it off. Just the sound of that TV was probably the only company she had. I found that so very sad.

We once went to an elderly gentleman who was feeling unwell. When we entered his upstairs bedroom, the floorboards started crumbling under our feet. He reminded me of the guy in the animated film *Up,* in that his world was literally falling apart around him. I can only assume he'd been walking on the joists for years. One foot wrong and he was gone.

We introduced ourselves and asked what we could do for him. After ascertaining that he needed to go to hospital, we had a chat about his living conditions: 'It doesn't feel safe for you in here. Would you like us to talk to someone about your situation? They might be able to help.' He wasn't one of those stubborn old people who didn't think anything was wrong and refused to be told, he agreed with us 100 per cent. No one had offered him the support he needed, and he didn't have money to repair his floor-boards. We decided it was too dangerous to try and get him out ourselves, so called the fire service. They managed to do the job by making sure to walk on the joists, which wasn't easy.

During our chat, the guy told us that he played dom-inoes in his local. That gave his situation a different angle. It made me realise that just because someone you meet might seem to be getting along fine, that's not necessarily the case. They might be living in deprivation but be too proud to tell anyone.

———

We're called to a concern for welfare incident, which usu-ally means someone has triggered a medical alarm or a member of the public is worried about a neighbour. An elderly lady hasn't been seen for a long time, and a post-man has noticed letters and junk mail piling up inside the front door and flies on the inside of the windows. Understandably, the hulking police officer who arrived on the scene before us suspects the worst, which is why he stands back and waves us in, having managed to gain entry through the back door.

I've never seen so many flies in my life; we are literally

brushing them aside with our feet as we creep along the hallway. This place is like the world's scariest haunted house, although I can tell that once upon a time it would have been immaculate. There are nice paintings on the wall and expensive-looking ornaments on sideboards. But it clearly went to rack and ruin a long time ago. There are plates piled up in the sink, mounds of rubbish everywhere and it smells of rotting food and matter. And every time we pop our heads into a room, there is every chance we'll be greeted by the sight of a decomposing corpse.

Nothing in the kitchen. Nothing in the bathroom. Nothing in the living room. Nothing in the dining room. Which leaves only one more room downstairs. I open the door and we all peer in. We must look like the lads and lasses from *Scooby-Doo*. In bed is an old lady. She looks about 150. She's emaciated, not much more than skin and bones, but looks peaceful. Just as I'm thinking, *Is she dead?*, the woman sits bolt upright and bellows, 'What are you doing in my house?'

I'm not ashamed to say I nearly shit myself. The burly copper, who is armed response, almost jumps out of his skin and lets out an almighty scream. I'm surprised he doesn't shoot the lot of us. Now, that would be a story.

The woman doesn't immediately calm down.

'Why are you here? Who let you in?'

'We're really sorry, but there were letters piling up behind your door. We thought you might need some help. Would you like us to phone social services?'

'No, I don't need anybody's help. Get out of my house!'

The copper, having finally stopped quaking, taps me on the shoulder and says, 'Come and have a look at what I've just found . . .'

I follow him into the living room and on the wall is a Perspex box, covered in flies. Inside the box is a painting and mounted next to it is a letter of authenticity, confirming that the painting is an original Picasso. Jesus Christ. This is a bit of a departure from the artwork we normally see on patients' walls, which ranges from Lowry prints to posters of Bob Marley smoking a spliff.

We spend a bit more time with the lady and discover that the only family she has is a distant cousin at the other end of the country who she hasn't seen for thirty years and doesn't have a contact number for. We have no choice but to leave her in the state she's in. We can't forcibly remove her, because it's not against the law to live how she's living, nor is it a medical emergency. All we can really do is contact her GP and refer her to social services, although we also make ourselves useful by doing a bit of cleaning and taking some rubbish out.

I did a bit of research on the Picasso and discovered it was part of a series. The last one sold at auction for millions of pounds. What does that say about money? Last I heard, the lady was still with us, lying in that bed, day after day, night after night, with not a friend in the world. She had all the money she ever needed but not the love and care. It's a sad story we'll probably never know in its entirety. If it has a silver lining, it's that her long-lost cousin has a lovely surprise coming to him.

Seeing things like that on a weekly basis changes a person. There are far too many jobs that make me think, *This is not what I signed up for.* Things that make me despair of society. I've been out to a homeless person who died in a public toilet. That cubicle was his final home and his deathbed. How are we allowing that to happen? Some argue that it's a lifestyle choice, but I find that hard to accept. I've attended people who have been beaten sense-less because they support a certain football team. Why would anyone do that? Grown men, fighting over a game. Stop the world, I want to get off.

———

Saturday night, and we get a call to a female intoxicated on the street. It sounds routine, as it almost always does. When we arrive on the scene, the woman is laid on the pavement and has wet herself. She's just down the road from the pub, so it's fairly safe to say she's had a few too many and collapsed on her way home. It's unorthodox to take people home these days because it carries risks. If, for example, they choke on their own vomit, we're in trouble. But once we manage to coax her address out of her – which is no mean feat in itself – we make the decision to run this woman back to her house and see if anyone is in.

We pull up outside, I jump out of the ambulance and my partner stays with her in the back. The house is in an affluent area and massive. The front door is slightly ajar and I can hear kids crying inside. I call out, 'Hello? Is anybody at home?' No answer. I'm a bit freaked out, so I run back to the ambulance and tell my partner what's going on. 'Are the kids all right?' she asks. Shit, the kids. I enter the house, while thinking someone is going to jump out on me with a baseball bat. Or a knife. I creep upstairs and find one kid, who must be about three, in bed. In another bed is a kid of about six months old, crying its eyes out and with a dog laid next to it, snoring contentedly.

I rush back to my partner, we lug the drunk lady inside, sling her on the sofa and phone for police assistance. While we wait for them to turn up, the baby just won't settle, so I make it a bottle and feed it. Thankfully, its nappy doesn't need changing, although with three kids of my own, I'm well used to it. About ten minutes later, this guy strolls in with a Chinese takeaway, bold as brass.

'What's going on here? Why are you in my house?'

'There's nobody at home with your kids, mate. And

we've just found your missus, drunk, lying in the street. Where have you been?'

'On a night out.'

'Who was supposed to be looking after the kids?'

'She was.'

Who leaves kids on their own and goes out and gets legless? But this guy has no shame at all. The police arrive as I'm winding the baby. They take some details, arrest the dad and take him away. The police find a number for the woman's mum and when she turns up, she's devastated. She's a lovely lady, and quite well-to-do. She takes her grandchildren home with her and leaves her daughter with us. When she finally regains consciousness, she's arrested as well: 'Surprise!'

Back in the ambulance, I feel strangely conflicted. It's obviously wrong what they did, but who was to blame? Did the man go out for a few beers and genuinely think his partner was at home looking after their kids? Or was it the other way around? Either way, clearly something is seriously wrong in that household. I can't help but think, *What happens next? What will become of these people?* At times like that I think, *This job is far deeper than I expected it to be.* Then another job comes on the screen and I get my head down and plough straight on.

———

It's not always the most dramatic jobs that stick in the memory. I once went out to a fella in his eighties who had taken an overdose before having second thoughts. He had a big house with a nice car parked out the front and was obviously a very successful man. But his wife had recently died and he couldn't stand the loneliness. On the way to hospital, he said to me, 'I don't know why I'm here. I've got no kids, no friends and I don't want to do this any more.'

What I usually say to someone in that situation is, 'Suicide is a permanent solution to a short-term problem.' But this case was a little bit different, because of his age. I explained that there were support groups out there, as well as societies and clubs where he could meet new people. I told him that it could be the first day of the rest of his life. It might sound trite, but what else could I do except try to give an old man hope in his hour of need?

I see so many people who are not really living but just clinging on by their fingertips, with no one to take their arm and lift them back up. I've seen couples in their nineties, with no family or friends, struggling to care for each other without any outside support. I've seen unwashed kids wearing no clothes running around dilapidated houses with ashtrays piled almost as high as the dishes in the kitchen sink.

Sometimes I think, *Who am I to judge?* The lines are often blurred between lifestyle choices and neglect. But sometimes I feel I have no choice but to refer patients to the relevant authorities. Even that process can prove frustrating, because after we've filled in the forms, we rarely hear anything back. Not only do we not know if we did the right thing, we don't know if it was even investigated. All we can do is cross our fingers.

Ambulance workers don't have time to get too philosophical about the things they see. But we do become very cynical. At least I have. I used to think I was a good Christian. I still hope there is something after death and I sent my children to a Christian school because I like the values the religion teaches. But the more you do my job, the less inclined you are to believe in a higher being. What kind of God would allow a child to die an agonising death from bone cancer? Or of neglect?

———

I have had the odd God conversation in the ambulance station, and you'll find that most people err on the side of science. Doctors and specialists can't work miracles in the biblical sense, but they work medical miracles every second of every day. I've never seen Jesus, but I have seen a percutaneous coronary intervention, which is essentially heart surgery done through a vein. No more being laid up for a month, you're out in a couple of days and back in the gym a few weeks later.

So until Jesus shows his face, I'll continue to believe in the evolved genius of humankind. And if I die, turn up at the pearly gates and they don't admit me, I'll get the police to knock them in.

8

Picking Up the Pieces

Ambulance clinicians are Jacks of all trades and masters of none. To extend the analogy, we're like the handyman you might call to unblock your drain or fix a leak. They're important jobs that need doing now, and a handyman is likely to be pretty good at them. But you wouldn't get him in to rewire your whole house, just as you wouldn't get an ambulance person in to rewire your brain. (Just to confirm, ambulance people are not – I repeat NOT – qualified to unblock your drain or fix a leak. We're busy enough as it is.)

When I started out on the road, I had a bit of an inferiority complex, because I hadn't been trained for stuff I'd been tasked to do. I assumed the doctors and specialists would look down on me, because that lot are trained for the best part of a decade. But I soon learned that when things get a bit sticky in a doctor's surgery and they need urgent medical assistance, they often call us.

We do a lot of picking up of pieces, sometimes literally. I've been called out to a doctor's surgery when a patient was taken acutely unwell. The doctor was clearly taken aback by this chap's medical condition, and it's safe to say that GPs aren't as used to dealing with that kind of stuff as us ambulance folk. He was very relieved to see us. So was the patient, as well as being slightly perplexed. Doctors and specialists understand that their game is their game, and our game is our game. And most ambulance workers are pretty good at it.

But there are times when I cease being an ambulance person and become a de facto carer, which is when my inferiority complex returns, because it's work that takes me miles out of my comfort zone. I sometimes attend terminally ill patients, who have called for an ambulance because they know they are about to die. One shift, I attended a 32-year-old lady who had been diagnosed with terminal cancer. Her organs had started to fail and I had no choice but to say, 'I think you're reaching the next stage.' She didn't want to remain at home because she had young children. And we didn't want to take her into A&E, because that didn't seem like the right place for her at all. So we phoned the local hospice, who mercifully agreed to take her in.

One of the most delicate jobs an ambulance person can do is remove a dying patient from their house while their family looks on. So it didn't matter how many jobs were waiting, we were going to take our time, because that's what this lady and her family deserved. We were in her house for what seemed like hours, readying her to leave for the final time. We can't make those experiences enjoyable, and we can't change the outcome, but we can try to make it as comfortable as possible. We tried to make it seem like what we were doing was nothing out of the ordinary, while giving the impression that nothing else mattered. Which, at that moment in time, it didn't.

We made sure to involve the patient in all our decisions, as if she was marshalling the process, rather than us. That meant not saying a great deal, unless we had to. But we weren't just there to support the patient – although she was our priority – we were there to support her family. That meant making the woman's husband and kids part of the process as well, so that they didn't feel like spare parts or they were getting in the way. We got the kids to help assemble the stretcher, so that they felt like they were helping their mum. And we lifted them up one by one, so that they could give her a kiss and a cuddle.

Daft as it might sound, a bit of humour is always welcome in such situations. At one point, the lady pointed to a window and said, 'I must give them a clean when I get back.' That showed incredible self-awareness: not only was it a coping mechanism, she was also trying to make the situation more tolerable for everyone else, including us.

On the way out, I noticed the lady looking around, taking it all in. We put her in the back of the ambulance as gently as we could, while feeling terrible that we were taking those poor kids' mum away to die. Before I jumped in the front, I said to her, 'Is there anything else we can do for you?' The lady said no, and thanked us for making the situation more bearable for her family. Those few words were better than any Christmas bonus. I held her hand for a moment and she gave me a weak smile. A slight squeeze of the fingers can say more than a thousand words. I wonder how many strangers' hands I've held.

Another time, we walked into a guy's house and the first thing he said was, 'Listen, I've been diagnosed with terminal cancer, I'm short of breath and I don't feel at all well. I think I'm dying, but I do not want resuscitating.' He conveyed his wishes quite strongly but didn't have a DNAR (do not attempt resuscitation) order in place. That was a conundrum. He was going to die and he wanted to die. But was he sufficiently sound of mind to make the decision for us to let him die? That was key, because if we agreed not to resuscitate him and it was later decided that he was not sufficiently sound of mind, we could have been in all sorts of legal bother.

We got on the phone to our senior bosses and asked a GP to attend, so that he could hopefully write out a DNAR. But now the question was, would the GP make it in time? And if he didn't arrive before the patient stopped breathing, where did we stand legally? The patient did indeed stop breathing before the GP arrived. Thankfully, several members of the patient's family were present, so we were able to ask them what they thought we should do. They were all in agreement that he shouldn't be resuscitated, so we made him comfortable and he passed away peacefully. Five minutes later, the GP knocked on the front door.

We kept the flurry of phone calls away from the patient and his family, but it still wasn't a particularly stress-free end for him – a couple of ambulance workers scrabbling around trying to get permission to let him die as he wanted. Given that his family were in attendance, he should have been able to say, 'I don't want to be resuscitated', end of story. It didn't sit right with me that his request was queried simply because he hadn't filled out a form.

The other side of the argument is that another family member not present might have put in a complaint that we didn't try to resuscitate. That can lead to a knock on the door from the police and a conviction for gross negligence. Ambulance people are often unsure if they're doing the right thing by the patient while adhering to the rules, because they don't always align exactly.

———

I spend a lot of time in care homes, for the obvious reason that the elderly are most likely to need my help. Some care homes are great, some are not so great. One place I go to has bingo most days, all sorts of activities and a piano, which they all sit around singing songs. It's more like a social club than a care home, I could manage a week in there myself. But there are other care homes that are little more than storehouses where the elderly are sent to spend the final years of their lives. The atmosphere can be quite sombre and you really feel for these people. If you put your dog in kennels, you expect the staff to give them stimulation. But that doesn't seem to be a priority in some of these places. Thankfully, the Care Quality Commission, established in 2008, has seen to it that a lot of the worst care homes be closed down. But some pretty bad ones remain.

We have an ageing population, but the country doesn't seem to have planned for it properly. There is not enough social care, which means elderly people who don't need urgent medical help are being taken to hospital because it's unsafe for them to remain at home. Add an overstretched GP service into the mix, and it means ambulance people are spending more and more of their time in elderly people's living rooms and A&E has become a fallback option. I'll often find myself thinking, *If there was better social care available, we could be dealing with someone who desperately needs us.* But services are slowly improving and, regardless, sitting and chatting with the elderly is one of the best parts of the job and makes me feel like I'm really doing something to help someone in need. I'd much rather be there than at a nightclub, especially as I love tea and custard creams.

Sometimes, we'll go to a job and it will quickly become apparent that an elderly person is simply lonely and wants some company for an hour. And even if we decide that their condition isn't serious enough for us to take them to hospital, we still spend time with them in order to reassure them. We might also arrange an appointment with their GP or refer them to a charity like Age UK, who will try to provide them with the social contact they need.

I've been to elderly people who have been unable to get out of their chair. Is it an emergency? Not really. Can we leave them stuck in their chair? Of course not. But if there is nothing medically wrong with them, it's a job a carer could be doing. Home carers do a wonderful job – popping in to massage an elderly lady's legs, cutting her toenails, checking that chesty cough hasn't developed into some-thing more worrying. And occupational therapists pimp up chairs and customise bedrooms and bathrooms. It's all about putting in place preventive measures so that people don't get stuck in their chair or bed, or fall down the stairs or in the shower. The only problem is, some people slip through the net.

Most home carers and carers in residential homes do an incredible job. I can't begin to imagine how difficult it must be to deliver care to people with all manner of debilitating illnesses. They do a lot of lifting and turning, a lot of wiping backsides and changing soiled sheets. They also deal with a lot of people with dementia, which can make them difficult to manage. On top of all that, they get to know their patients really well, before watching them disintegrate and die. But these carers are almost impossible to faze and have such a lovely, tender manner. And what do we pay these heroes, who do one of the most important jobs in the world? Not much more than the minimum wage.

For all the great work our carers do, I sometimes think our elderly people are written off too quickly. I was on a day off (we do have them) when my wife's dad called to say her nan had had a stroke. The doctor said she was going to die within twenty-four hours, so they needed to come and say their goodbyes.

Off we popped to the care home, but the whole way there I was thinking, *How does he know she's going to die within the next twenty-four hours?* In the ambulance service, we don't write someone off who's had a stroke and wait for them to die, we treat them. I couldn't compute it. But I had a little word with myself, to remind myself I wasn't on shift: *Don't walk in being Billy Big Bollocks, leave the work hut by the door. Just keep your mouth shut . . .*

As soon as I walked into her room, I could see that she hadn't had a stroke. A stroke has very specific symptoms: a patient will have facial weakness, meaning they won't be able to smile and/or their mouth or eye will be drooping; their speech might be slurred and they might not be able to understand you; they might not be able to raise their arms. You don't really need to be a medical person to know what a stroke looks like, and this doctor was way off the mark. The poor woman was rolling around on the bed, breathing really fast. Her temperature was through the roof. It was obvious she had an infection.

When the doctor finally turned up, I said, 'What makes you think she's had a stroke? I think she should be in hospital.' He replied, 'I think she should remain here and be allowed to die in peace.' I'm all for letting people die in peace if there's nothing more we can do for them, but I was absolutely certain that my wife's nan was treatable. So I phoned an ambulance, explaining, 'Look, this doctor wants to leave her to die, but I think she's got sepsis.' (Sepsis is a serious complication of an infection and needs to be treated as quickly as possible.)

As soon as my colleagues saw her, they agreed with my diagnosis. They stuck her in the ambulance, switched on the blues and twos and whisked her off to hospital. The doctor took one look at her and diagnosed sepsis. At first she responded to treatment, but her organs failed and she died a couple of days later. Had her doctor not waited twelve hours, I believe she might have survived.

While I have enormous respect for anyone who works as a medical professional, and sympathy for the fact they live in constant fear of being complained about, I had no hesitation in reporting this doctor to the General Medical Council. Perhaps some people might have thought, *You know what? She was old and on her way out anyway, it's not worth the hassle.* But I wasn't having it.

It made me look at complainants in a different light. Some complaints are petty and put medical professionals through an awful lot of stress for no reason, because any complaint is taken seriously. But medical professionals are human, so they do make mistakes. In this case, the doctor got suspended and he resigned before his hearing could take place.

But of all the things I've seen in my time in the ambulance service, hospices are the most heart-wrenching. Not just because they're full of dying people, but also because of the quite wonderful staff who care for them. Hospices care for 200,000 people a year but are charities, so rely on tens of thousands of volunteers and fundraisers to survive. On average, adult hospices receive a third of their funding from the state, children's hospices only about 15 per cent. But if it weren't for hospices, what would happen to the people who rely on their care? Would they be in A&E instead? That doesn't even bear thinking about.

Staff in any hospice, all of them criminally underpaid and many of them paid nothing, must be incredibly resilient. Staff in children's hospices must be some of the most resilient people on the planet. It must be an incredibly tough job, but very rewarding at the same time. It's a huge responsibility, but there can't be many jobs more worthy than making someone's last moments on earth as comfortable as possible and providing them with a dignified death, while also ensuring that the situation is as palatable as possible for their family.

9

MOMENTS OF MADNESS

Usually when we turn up to a job, the patient and their loved ones are very relieved to see me, as you might expect. A patient might have had a heart attack and their wife or husband won't have a clue what's going on and what to do about it. We can provide them with answers and hopefully solve their problem, or at least deliver them to people who can. As such, people are normally quite respectful. When people aren't respectful, there are two common denominators: drugs and alcohol. Though, in a weird way, it's comforting that it might have taken twelve pints of Stella and five shots of sambuca to convince someone that I'm not their guardian angel, but a colossal idiot who deserves to be abused or attacked.

It's a sunny summer afternoon, and we're called to a man intoxicated and collapsed on the street. He's part of a stag party which has been travelling on a coach for three or four hours, getting bang on the booze. When the coach parks up, this bloke steps off, gets a blast of fresh air, topples straight over and smashes his head on the pavement. One of his mates phones 999 and we get the shout.

My partner is wheeling (driving the ambulance), so it's my turn for healing (attending the patient). I crouch over this bloke and say, 'Hiya, mate, it's the ambulance. Can you hear me?' And this bloke responds with an uppercut to my chin, delivered from a prone position. It only grazes me, so it doesn't particularly hurt. And maybe he's suddenly come round, felt someone prodding him in the chest, got spooked and lashed out. But still.

We have control of the situation, but this bloke's mates start getting a bit gobby. There are about twenty of them stood around us, all offering advice on what we should and shouldn't be doing, while arguing with each other. And when you've just been punched and people are getting a bit gobby, it's time to press the emergency button on our radio – or, as we call it, the 'tits-up button'. Luckily, it's match day, so having pressed the tits-up button, four riot vans come screaming from every direction, their appearance bringing the gobbiness to an instant halt. Had it not been match day, we might have been in trouble. As it is, my assailant is dragged to his feet, arrested, chucked in the back of a van and whisked off to the police station. He's been in town for about twenty minutes, fallen over drunk, whacked an ambulanceman, been nicked and locked in a cell. It's like a rubbish version of *The Hangover*. The following morning, he appears in court and is fined 25 quid. That'll learn him.

Sometimes people will blame their unruly and embarrassing behaviour on their drink being spiked. We'll turn up to a patient paralytic on the pavement and their mates will say, 'I don't know what's happened. This isn't like Jane, she can normally drink a lot more than this.' What they won't mention is that Jane has necked five shots on top of a bottle of Prosecco, hasn't eaten since breakfast and only had three hours' sleep the previous night. There is a genuine problem of women having their drinks spiked with Rohypnol in bars and clubs (although that's not something I've ever had to deal with), but that's not usually what's happened. And drug dealers aren't noted for their generosity, so it's highly unlikely they're dropping their produce into random people's drinks. That doesn't make much business sense.

When you see someone crashing around on the street, you probably assume they're drunk or on drugs. But that's not necessarily the case. One day, a job came on the screen: MALE FITTING. That's not uncommon and there are a few possible reasons, including epilepsy or withdrawal from alcohol.

When me and Paul arrived on the scene, which was on a busy street, the guy had stopped fitting but was still flat on his back and out of it. We gave him a shot of oxygen, I grabbed the stretcher and just as we were about to lift him on it, he suddenly woke up and sprung to his feet. He tried to punch us, then tried to start a fight with a young couple walking past with their kids. And, had we not pulled him out of the road, he might have been mown down by a double-decker bus. We quickly concluded that he was having a postictal episode, which is when confusion kicks in after you wake up from a fit and you slip into fight or flight mode.

We requested the police attend, but they don't just appear out of thin air. And while the police were en route, we were the only people on the scene wearing uniforms, having arrived in a vehicle with sirens blaring and flashing blue lights. As such, people expected us to do something. This was a no-win situation. Our rules probably say we should have legged it, but we couldn't just stand by and let this bloke run amok. And forget the fact that we were ambulance people, we had a responsibility as citizens to stop this bloke hurting himself or anyone else.

He swung at us again, me and Paul both grabbed him and we all ended up in a big heap on the floor. Now we were in a particularly sticky spot. Some people told us to leave him alone and stop pinning him down. Other people were shouting, 'You're supposed to be ambulancemen, not the police.' We weren't really in a position to explain that he was in a postictal state and that what tends to occur with these types of episodes are auditory and visual hallucinations, delusions, paranoia and aggression. We just about had enough breath to explain that we were actually trying to help him. The icing on the cake would have been if someone had pulled out their phone and started filming us. That wouldn't have looked good on social media, because people tend to put two and two together and get five. If people had seen two ambulancemen lying on top of a patient in the street, they would have put two and two together and got five. The public aren't interested in finding out the details, they see a snapshot of a situation and jump to conclusions.

Just as the police arrived, the guy suddenly came to, as if a switch had been flicked in his brain. And now he was back in the room, he was absolutely mortified. He had nothing to apologise for, because he didn't know what he was doing. Meanwhile, Paul announced that he had injured his knee. He could barely walk to the ambulance and ended up off work for six months with a torn meniscus. It could have been worse. If it had been the patient who busted his knee instead of Paul, we could have been in serious trouble. As it was, our bosses were not impressed: 'You've hurt your knee restraining someone? What were you bloody thinking? You're not supposed to be restraining anyone!'

———

My home patch on a Friday and Saturday night is often described by the media as 'a warzone'. But that's what they want it to be, because it's a story that sells. When they filmed *999: What's Your Emergency?*, they hardly showed any of the routine stuff, like attending an elderly man who had died in his sleep or a toddler with a fever. Mostly, they showed aggressive lads covered in blood and paralytic girls in very short skirts falling over and passing out. It was a bit soul-destroying, not only because it didn't show us doing our jobs to the best of our abilities, but also because it conveyed the town in such a bad light. The town and its people didn't deserve that, so we felt a bit stitched-up.

Generally speaking, the town is a lovely place for families to visit. Yes, it caters for stag and hen dos, which means we have a lot of people out at weekends drinking more than they would normally. But most people, even with a few drinks inside them, just want to have a good time, some fun and frolics. They're friendly and have a bit of a laugh with us when we arrive on scene. Sometimes girls will lift their tops and flash us their breasts. Or, on a bad night, they'll just give us a wave.

Truthfully, mostly on a weekend it's more mundane

stuff we deal with: people walking in front of cars, getting lost on the way home and freezing on a bench, attempting a caterpillar on the dancefloor and landing on their face. So to say it's a warzone out there, or 'carnage', is an exaggeration. It's not like we're being pelted with bottles and having drinks poured over our heads.

Fun and frolics will occasionally give way to something more sinister, like people screaming at each other in the street or scrapping on the pavement, and occasionally someone ends up injured. Nine times out of ten, the injury will be a fractured cheekbone or a broken eye socket and we'll need to take them to hospital for an x-ray. But sometimes it's worse.

One balmy summer's evening – the sort of evening that makes me glad to be doing the job – we are called to an altercation between a couple of punters in a pub. One bloke mistakenly thought this other bloke had been mithering his sister and whacked him on their way out. Whether it was the punch or his head bouncing off the pavement that did the damage is arguable, but the victim of the assault is bleeding heavily and critically ill when we get there. We do what we can, but he passes away a couple of days later. One man dead and another man behind bars, all because of a moment of madness.

Someone who's not in the ambulance service might go years without seeing a fight in a pub, but I might attend the aftermath of five pub brawls in a week. So doing my job has made me hyper-sensitive. When I'm out socially, I find myself profiling people: judging how drunk they are, whether they're on drugs, what kind of mood they're in, whether they're happy or angry, whether they're about to flip. If I see people having a disagreement in a pub, I'm on edge, weighing up possible outcomes. I've been to so many fights where an innocent bystander has been caught in the middle, and I don't want that to happen to a friend or family member. I'm also thinking, *Lads, just calm down a bit, or you might do something stupid that will destroy both your lives.*

It isn't just drunks and grown men fighting over a game of football that eat into an ambulance person's time that would be better spent treating someone's poor gran who has fallen down the stairs. Drugs are also a major problem. It's very rare for us to treat someone with a complication from taking 'recreational' drugs, such as marijuana, cocaine or ecstasy – although that's not the same as saying they're safe. We do, however, see more heroin overdoses.

The youngest victim of a heroin overdose I treated was seventeen. He was bleeding out of every orifice, so that the back of the ambulance looked like an abattoir. We do carry a drug, naloxone, that can reverse the effects. In America, they administer it as a nasal spray; we inject it (although it's not like that scene in *Pulp Fiction* where John

111

Travolta smashes a needle into Uma Thurman's chest, it's just a little injection in the patient's arm). Usually when we administer it, the patient springs back to life. You'd think they'd be thankful, but they're normally angry that you've ruined their fix. And most of the time they'll refuse to go with you to the hospital. I'll feel like saying to them, 'Come on mate, you weren't breathing a few seconds ago.' But naloxone didn't work for this kid – we thought because the heroin he'd taken was laced with rat poison, which thins the blood. Whatever the reason, try as we might, we couldn't get him breathing again and he was pronounced dead shortly after arriving at hospital.

People will do anything to block out the horrible realities of their existence. But while I understand why people become dependent on drugs, I do find myself wondering what the authorities are doing to try to stop it happening. I see charities trying to help these people, but we shouldn't really need charities to take up the slack. You can debate whose responsibility it is all you like, but when you're dealing with a dead person who spent his final hours in a public toilet, you realise something desperately needs to be done. Sometimes I feel more like a dustman than an ambulanceman: people are tossed on the street, I sweep them up and everything goes on as before.

You wouldn't believe how some of your fellow humans meet their end. A very senior colleague was called to a heroin overdose: two guys had taken a hit, gone to wherever they go to, and when one of them came to, he found his mate had gone blue. As they say in the drug world, he had 'gone over'. That's not uncommon, because heroin is a respiratory suppressant, which is a fancy way of saying it stops you breathing. And if you stop breathing for too long, you'll go into a cardiac arrest and die.

This bloke was scared to phone an ambulance, because he thought the crew would see the drugs and call the police. It doesn't actually work like that, mainly because of patient confidentiality, but also because we don't want to deter people from calling in that situation. The exception is when someone dies. Anyway, this bloke panicked and decided to take things into his own hands. He'd obviously seen a few episodes of *Casualty* and someone using a defibrillator, and thought, *That looks easy enough*. So he'd dismantled a lamp and attempted to resuscitate his mate with two bare wires. It did not have the desired effect and electrocuted his mate instead. So listen up you crazy kids: if one of your mates has a heroin overdose, phone the professionals.

Another drug that seems to be all the rage at the minute is spice, which is a plant-based mix of herbs laced with synthetic chemicals and often far stronger than cannabis. It's particularly popular among homeless people because it's so cheap. And you'll know if a homeless person has smoked too much of it, because they'll be standing there like a statue, often bent double. You can take a trip into oblivion for less than a fiver's worth of spice, which is exactly why they take it. But when you could still buy spice over the counter (it was made illegal in 2016), we were dealing with people with families and jobs, who took it thinking it was harmless fun.

One guy was on holiday with his family. He was a weed smoker, but because he didn't know any dealers in the area, he bought some spice from a shop. A few hours after smoking it, he tried to eat his wife and kids. You read that correctly. He was chasing them around the hotel room, trying to take chunks out of them. It took eight policemen to hold him down. He wasn't a big guy, but he was like Popeye just after he'd had his spinach.

Another victim of spice I encountered was a young woman who was persuaded by a friend to try it on a night out. When she crossed my path, she was being transferred from A&E to psychiatric care. It had caused a chemical imbalance in her brain, so that she didn't know who she was, where she was or what she was seeing. A nurse told me that it could take weeks, months or years for her to return to normal. Or maybe she never would. She was a good-looking, otherwise sensible girl with a good job working for the council, but a bit of spice on a Saturday night out had sent her life into a sudden tailspin.

———

I've never attended anyone who's been shot and stabbings are very rare, even though they seem to be all the rage in other parts of the country. Most stabbings on my patch are domestic – someone grabbing a knife from the kitchen, as happened to me. Although, don't get me wrong, stabbings, whatever the circumstance, are not nice to deal with, especially if we arrive before the police. Not only is it messy and pressurised work, there will often be at least one other very upset person on the scene. So while we're administering complicated treatment to the patient, we're also trying to keep that other person calm. In addition, we're thinking, *I wonder where the attacker has gone*. We just have to hope they made their escape long before we got there. But you never know. People often stab to kill, and if someone ever decided to come back and finish the job, we'd only have our fists to defend ourselves with.

I went to a chap once who had fallen off his push-bike and was laid out on the pavement. Despite being unconscious, his feet were still pedalling, which was undeniably spooky. We didn't know what was wrong with him, because he didn't have any obvious injuries. But when we lifted his jumper up to get to his chest, we found a set of bolt cutters and a big knife in his pocket. But even though this kid had obviously been up to no good, we still did our very best to help him, as did the nurses, doctors and specialists at the hospital. In the case of this chap, it wasn't enough, because he died of a bleed to the brain.

For all the overdose victims I've treated in drug dens and toilets, I've also treated middle-class people who had taken overdoses in comfortable homes. I've also been out to an end-stage alcoholic who happened to be a GP. Nobody is immune. One of the things I love about the NHS is that whoever you are and wherever you're from, you have a right to the very best treatment the NHS can offer. Whether a patient lives in a house whose floors stick to my feet or whose carpet is 6 inches deep, they deserve the same care and they get the same care. Accidents and illness don't discriminate, so neither do we.

10

FIND A BLOODY DOCK LEAF

People always ask me about the weirdest injuries I've seen. Seconds later they'll be asking about bizarre sex injuries. That's normally the way it pans out. Well, I once went out to a man who claimed he was making love to his missus and, to use his exact words, had 'snapped his knob'. We turned up, knocked on his door, asked very few questions and whisked him off to hospital. If a man says he's snapped his knob, I'm taking his word for it: 'Broke your knob? On you get.' Unless he was bleeding to death, I wasn't going to start inspecting it. Snapped knobs are not my area of expertise. What do you do with a snapped knob? Stick a plaster cast on it?

I've also been out to a fair few snapped banjo strings – or, more correctly, frenulums – which are the small tags of skin between the foreskin and the shaft of a penis. A snapped banjo string can cause major panic, because one minute someone might be making sweet love, the next the sheets are covered in claret. Usually by the time we've arrived on the scene, the bleeding has stopped. If it hasn't, we'll tell the patient to wrap their old chap in a tea towel and hop on the ambulance. I must have missed that day in training.

I was eighteen years old, wet behind the ears, having just started work in the ambulance control room. A call came in, I got the guy to confirm his address and phone number and asked him what seemed to be the problem. The guy hesitated. He then started mumbling, so that I couldn't understand him. So I asked him to tell me again, but this time clearer. A long pause. Then he began: 'Well ... I've just got out of the shower, slipped, fallen down the stairs, landed on top of the hoover, somehow turned it on and now my penis is stuck.'

My immediate thought was, *Is this bloke taking the mick?* But we sent an ambulance to his house. To be fair to the bloke, it's not as if he could have jumped in a taxi with a Dyson hanging off his John Thomas. I can't remember how it turned out for this chap, but I assume they managed to free him. If not, he can't be difficult to spot.

It's not uncommon for someone to present themselves at A&E with all sorts of objects stuck in their nether regions. The staff are obviously discreet and try to be rational about it: it's the twenty-first century, people have sex toys and sometimes things get out of hand. But while most people like to keep their tales of experimentation gone wrong under wraps, one brave lady from Liverpool (a mother of one, no less) went public a few years ago, telling newspapers that she got a vibrator stuck up her backside in the throes of passion and that her boyfriend was unable to remove it, even with a fork handle (why?) and a pair of barbeque tongs (makes far more sense). Eventually, the woman went to hospital and a surgeon removed the (still buzzing) vibrator, before offering it to her as a keepsake. She declined. I'd love to know how she explained her absence to her daughter.

Sometimes there are stories that blow the mind of even veteran medical professionals. A colleague of mine once went out to a guy who had inserted a dildo that was so long, it was almost coming out of his mouth. On the way there, my colleague was thinking, *Why would he phone an ambulance? Why not just take himself to hospital?* When he arrived, he realised why.

For hours, this guy had been trying to extricate this dildo, to no avail. It's not really the sort of thing Ask Jeeves will have the answer to on the internet, although I'm sure people have asked. He'd had his hand up there, as if he was playing a more risqué version of the claw crane game you see in seaside arcades. And when that had failed (as the claw crane game usually does), he'd decided to have a root around with one of those big serving spoons dinner ladies use in schools. He had caused himself quite major trauma, was bleeding heavily and my colleague had to take him in for major surgery.

Clearly, the chap with the giant dildo up his bum desperately needed the NHS's help. But you wouldn't believe some of the nonsense ambulance people get sent to. Ask any ambulance person about the 111 helpline and they'll give you a wry smile or raise an eyebrow. NHS 111 is partly staffed by non-clinicians with a checklist of questions, and they are quite risk-averse. I don't blame the call handlers, because they're doing an incredibly tough job. And the computer asks a lot of leading questions, such as, 'Do you have chest pains? Are you coughing a lot?' If the answer is, 'Oh, aye, I am feeling a bit chesty, and I'm coughing my head off,' an ambulance will likely be sent.

A patient might have to wait a month for an appointment with their GP. And if the GP can't find a solution to the problem, they'll want to refer it to a specialist. But there might be a three-month wait to see a specialist, so either the GP or the patient will end up phoning 999 and an ambulance will be sent to whisk them to A&E. To compound the problem, patients are no longer able to make appointments out of hours, so they'll be asked to phone 111 instead.

Someone will pop into an NHS walk-in centre with a relatively minor ailment and a nurse or doctor will insist they go to hospital. The person will say, 'Oh. Really? Okay, I've got my car outside.' And the nurse or doctor will say, 'No, we'll call you an ambulance.' I've seen it happen. In the old days, a nurse or doctor would have relied far more on their experience and clinical skills, so that there were a lot more diagnoses of 'You'll be all right.'

How often do you hear the advice, 'Don't call for an ambulance unless you absolutely need it'? But it's amazing how many women go into labour, still with plenty of time to spare, and call us to take them in to hospital. We call it 'maternataxi'. We turn up and they say, 'We haven't got any money for a cab.' Some women are genuinely skint, but others are perfectly well off. It's like they've only just noticed they're pregnant. It's also not uncommon to arrive at the hospital and for the patient to jump out of the back of the ambulance and spark up a cigarette. I feel like saying, 'Are you taking the piss?' They've phoned 999, we've steamed over to their house, taken them in and they're well enough to stop off for a leisurely smoke before going into A&E.

Off the top of my head, I've heard of someone wanting an ambulance to be sent to resuscitate a dead pigeon, help find someone's trousers, deal with a hedgehog in a garden, treat someone whose feet were bleeding from wearing new shoes and fix a dislodged (false) fingernail. The media loves compiling lists of ridiculous 999 calls, and they would be funny if they weren't such a pain in the arse.

And not all of the daftness gets filtered out. I've been out to someone who phoned 111 to report that his plaster cast was making his arm itchy. You can't stop people from calling, all you can do is provide a service that filters out the time-wasters. As mad as phoning 111 to report an itchy arm is, the fact that we ended up at his house wasn't really his fault, it was the fault of the system and how the questions were answered. What did I say when I turned up at Itchy's house? I pinned him to the floor and broke his other arm. Nah. I smiled as usual, was nice and chipper, told him that everything was going to be okay and suggested he be a brave soldier and wait for the itch to go away. Thanks for calling 111! Had I not been nice and polite, he might have complained about my attitude.

How long can the NHS continue sending ambulances out to patients who have diarrhoea or who have been sick a couple of times? At what point will it say enough is enough? Maybe we should have a system whereby people pay a smallish fee at the point of use. Not a lot, but enough to put people off. Then again, 20 quid to one person is a drop in the ocean, while to another it's their kids' dinner budget for the week.

Rather than reduce the load on the ambulance service, the internet has made it worse. The internet is all-knowing, but it is so vast that it often throws up more questions than answers. While an older person is likely to have a more common sense and less dramatic reaction to going down with an illness (as well as drive themselves or a friend or family member to hospital) a younger person might find themselves with a spot of man flu, go on Dr Google and ten minutes later they'll have convinced themselves that their headache is actually a brain tumour or they've got nine different diseases and only three days to live.

I suspect younger people are also less likely to understand what the emergency services are for, and they've become accustomed to getting what they want at the drop of a hat, twenty-four hours a day, seven days a week, however urgent their need. What they need to understand is, the ambulance service does not operate along the same lines as a pizza delivery company. Well, sometimes it does. But it shouldn't.

There is also the issue of people trying to nick a few quid from insurance claims. Once, me and my partner were on our way to a bog-standard job when we got flagged down by a bus driver who was standing next to a double-decker that had had a minor prang with a car. I called the control room and they dispatched a different crew to the other job. I jumped out of the ambulance and the first thing I said to the bus driver was, 'Is everyone okay?' The bus driver replied, 'I think so. But I'll just go and make sure.'

We hopped on the bus, the driver asked if anyone was hurt and what happened next was like that scene from *Spartacus*: one hand went up and soon everyone had their hand up. So now I had fifty-two 'patients' all complaining of neck pain. Or, as we call it in the trade, 'whipcash'.

We were on the scene for hours, taking names and addresses and writing down fifty-two different versions of the same story, some far more dramatic than others. No one let on that it was all a con, but they knew that we knew. We could see it in each other's eyes. What could we say? 'Come on. You're taking the mick. There's nothing wrong with you!' Instead, they went on their merry way, sent the paperwork off to the relevant people, along with a letter explaining that they'd been in a bus crash and had to be assessed by an ambulance person, and maybe got some compensation out of it.

Mobile phones also play their part. Before mobiles, if someone saw a bloke slumped in the street, looking like he might need assistance, they might ask him if he was okay, or, far more likely, walk on by. If someone was punched outside a pub, they'd go home and put some ice on their eye. Now, you get a lot of people phoning 999 and saying stuff like, 'I've just driven past someone in the doorway of a shop and he didn't look very well. Could you send an ambulance?' It's lovely that people are looking out for their fellow human beings, but it means we get sent to a lot of situations that don't require us to be there. Don't get me wrong, I'm not discouraging people to call for help, but maybe it's worth asking the person in the shop doorway first.

One night, someone phoned to say they'd seen a man 'walking sideways like a crab'. It wasn't difficult to find him, because he was walking sideways like a crab. But the reason he was walking sideways like a crab was because he'd drunk about ten pints of strong European lager. I pointed him in the direction of the taxi rank, got on to the control room and shoehorned as many crab jokes into the conversation as I could: 'Yes, we tracked him down, although he was a bit nippy. He's scuttled off now. Little bit shellfish, didn't even say thank you . . .'

I've also been out to a nettle sting. No, I'm not making this up. This guy phoned 111, said he'd walked through some nettles and his legs hurt. All he needed to be told was, 'Get yourself down to your local chemist, buy some ointment, put it on the affected area and you'll be right as rain in no time.' Instead, the call was passed to us, which was a classic example of the problems with computer-generated responses to people's injuries and ailments. On the way to this guy's house, I still wanted to give him the benefit of the doubt. I said to my partner, 'All he did was

125

phone for advice, he probably doesn't even want us coming round.' My partner replied, 'Why would anyone phone 111 for advice about a nettle sting? Go out and find a bloody dock leaf!' He had a point.

The NHS has tried to find ways to combat the madness – just as the NHS tries to find ways to solve any problem thrown at it. Control rooms are now staffed with paramedics, nurses and even pharmacists, to whom less urgent calls are triaged. They might phone a caller back, reassess their situation and decide if there is an alternative to sending an ambulance. They might advise the caller to make their own way to hospital, or that they don't require treatment at all. We also have a special team whose job is to visit frequent callers and see if they can teach them to understand the difference between an ailment and a genuine emergency. That's good for the patient and good for the ambulance service, as is anything that helps takes the strain off.

Every ambulance station has its regular customers, the so-called 'frequent flyers'. An address will come on the screen and we know immediately that we're heading back to Fred's house on London Road. Some of the frequent flyers are genuinely ill and only call in an emergency. Others are after a hit of morphine or pain-relieving Entonox, more commonly known as gas and air. I suspect others look upon a trip to hospital in the back of an ambulance as a bit of excitement, a change from their usual humdrum existence.

————

As well as tying up someone in the control room for a couple of minutes, while they could be dealing with someone having a heart attack, each phone call costs the ambulance service about £7, so one person making hundreds of calls a year can cost thousands of pounds. I've heard of people getting hit with ambulance ASBOs, which means that if they call and it's discovered it's not an emergency, they can end up in prison. But these people are sometimes impossible to ignore. The rule of thumb is that if someone calls complaining of chest pains, we will send an ambulance. Certain callers know this, and you can bet your life that if we ever decided not to send an ambulance, the caller would be having a genuine heart attack.

People might assume ambulance people hold frequent flyers in contempt – at least those with nothing much physically wrong with them. But that's not necessarily the case. Some of them are mentally ill. For example, they might have Munchausen's syndrome, which means they'll pretend to be ill because they crave the fuzzy feeling of being looked after. Then there's fabricated or induced illness, which is when a parent will exaggerate or delib-erately cause symptoms of illness in their child. But a lot of the time, frequent flyers are simply lonely. I know that, because they sometimes tell me.

Like teachers, we shouldn't really have favourites. But we do. One lad called Barry used to phone all the time, with ailments ranging from chest pains to shortness of breath to whatever he could think of on the day. Barry had been raised in children's homes and supported by the state ever since. He had learning difficulties and while he knew that phoning us all the time was wrong, he couldn't grasp the severity of it.

He was a bit of a nuisance, but he was also a really nice guy who knew us all by name and made us laugh every time we went out to him. Barry had a wicked sense of humour. Once, I stalled the ambulance while he was in the back and he was roaring with laughter and slapping his knee, as if it was the funniest thing he'd ever seen. One Christmas, he brought out this wad of bank notes, gave them to us and said, 'Get your missus something nice.' Except they weren't bank notes, they were pieces of toilet paper printed to look like bank notes.

I once joked that we were going to remove the number nine button from his phone. He thought that was hilarious. The next time we went there, he told us that he'd hidden it. Sometimes we were quite stern with him – 'Seriously, Barry, you mustn't phone for an ambulance unless you really, really need one' – and he'd promise not to do it again. But we'd be round there a couple of weeks later. It was impossible to be mad at him. Barry was just lonely and wanted a chat, which he even admitted towards the end.

Some might argue that it's wrong to get too close to these people, that we're feeding their habit. But not everything is so black and white. And we're only human. If someone seems like a genuinely good person, we'll naturally be protective of them. And having witnessed their loneliness and desperation up close, we want things to get better for them once we've left the scene. But that's not always the case. Barry was a big drinker and smoker and died young. Quite a few ambulance staff and nurses went to his funeral. Had we not, no one would have been there. In death, as in life, we were his only friends.

11

A LACK OF RESPECT

Me and my partner are called to a male who has taken an overdose. Whenever anybody calls 999, it's the job of the dispatcher to assess if the scene might be volatile or dangerous for the ambulance people. It's often a tricky call to make, especially if the patient is calling for themselves, because they're highly unlikely to say, 'I'm not feeling too clever, but if you do send an ambulance round, I might try to fight them when they get here.' This particular call is deemed as non-violent, so off we trot, with hardly a care in the world.

On arrival at the scene, the front door is slightly ajar. I knock, but no one answers. That's not uncommon. I knock a second time and hear someone shout, 'Come in!' There is no one in the hallway, so I pop my head around the door of the living room. BOOM! Some unseen person punches me square in the face. I promptly hit the deck like a sack of spuds, but still have enough faculties to think, *What did he do that for?* We don't get taught self-defence by the ambulance service. We do get taught breakaway techniques (how to break free from an aggressor in a safe manner), but like any tools, they become rusty when you don't use them too often.

Luckily, my partner is right behind me and quickly incapacitates my assailant (using the approved techniques, obviously). Punchy soon pipes down, and we have no choice but to sit on top of him until the police arrive, because every time we release the pressure, he starts trying to hit us again.

It turns out this bloke is a regular caller, and the fact he's chinned me suggests he's high as a kite, although he might have a mental health or behavioural problem. Often, it's difficult to tell. The following day, a police officer calls to tell me that my assailant has been given a formal warning and ordered to pay me compensation: £20, to be paid in instalments. Every week for the next two years, 20p will land in my account. There's some more of that gallows humour I was talking about.

You have to be very versatile to work in the ambulance service. A GP has to adapt to each individual patient and a variety of cases, but normally in a controlled and comfortable environment. Frontline ambulance workers have to adapt to strangers, a bewildering variety of cases and our surroundings. One minute we might be chatting with an old lady in a lovely big house, the next we might be dealing with an overdose in a drug den, the next we might be dealing with someone who has been punched unconscious in a banging nightclub.

Because ambulance staff aren't equipped with body armour or weaponry, we have to rely on the gift of the gab to get us out of threatening situations, which is why most of my colleagues are very effective communicators. We also develop an acute sense of when to stay away.

On another occasion, me and my partner are called to a male with a shotgun, who is threatening to shoot the next person who comes around the corner. We get the gig because someone has decided it's a mental health case. But you could quite easily argue that while anyone who is threatening to commit a violent act is mentally ill, that doesn't mean they should be sending us in to deal with it instead of the police. We're lurking around the corner from this bloke's house when the Old Bill finally turn up. For all we know, he could have had an air rifle, but we aren't going to take any chances.

The copper asks us, 'Where is he then?'

'He's round the corner. But he's got a gun and is threatening to use it.'

'I'll go and have a look . . .'

This copper trots off and I turn to my mate and say, 'What an idiot.' All this officer has is a can of hairspray on his hip.

Thirty seconds later, the copper reappears out of breath and shouting, 'He's got a fucking gun!' I raise an eyebrow.

My colleague says, 'Yes mate, we just told you that.'

In the end, the police see sense and send an armed response team in.

When things go pear-shaped, sometimes we just have to hope right-minded members of the public have our back, because we can't be sure there will be immediate police assistance. We have a great working relationship with the police. There's a good deal of mutual empathy and a lot of crossover, at road traffic accidents, incidents of domestic violence and serious mental health jobs. For example, if someone is detained under Section 136 of the Mental Health Act, the police will travel in the back of our ambulance with the patient. That's not to say they're a criminal, but they are often a threat to themselves.

There is a mutual understanding that both services are run off their feet but will do anything to help each other. But police cuts haven't just affected the police and the public, they have had an adverse effect on the ambulance service. When there were a lot more police about, they'd readily come and help us when we needed it. But now, the police are so overstretched that when we press our tits-up button, we can't be sure we won't end up in a lengthy queue.

Our control room might send us to a potentially violent patient and ask us to carry out a DORA, which stands for Dynamic Operational Risk Assessment. But how can you assess how much of a risk that potentially violent person is unless you're face to face with him or her? And by that time, it might be too late.

There is more and more risk-taking creeping in. Nine times out of ten, the police are right not to send anyone. But it only takes that one time. I worry for the police as well. It can be a scary job, and they do the best with what they've got. And they must get frustrated with us, because sometimes they'll be waiting for hours for an ambulance to arrive and take a patient from them.

I'm terrified the time will come when someone in the ambulance service gets seriously hurt, or worse. According to figures from the trade union GMB, 72 per cent of ambulance workers have been physically assaulted while on duty. There were 14,000 attacks on ambulance workers between 2012 and 2018.

I've been reasonably lucky. I've been punched a few times and had snowballs thrown at my ambulance, which doesn't sound like much but isn't ideal when you're travelling at 70mph. But colleagues have been bitten, had bones broken and, in other parts of the country, stab wounds. I've heard of ambulance staff being taken hostage, attacked with samurai swords, having bricks and bottles thrown at them, blood spat at them by intravenous drug users and cars driven at them. I've even heard stories of ambulance workers being attacked and members of the public filming it on their phones rather than coming to their aid. Sexual assaults on ambulance workers are also more prevalent, including lewd remarks, verbal threats and indecent exposure.

Attacks on ambulances themselves have also gone up, including bottles and metal poles being thrown through windows and vehicles ransacked. There was even a phase of people nicking cylinders of pain-relieving Entonox from station stores and the back of ambulances, which they thought would give them a high. Unfortunately, our gas is mixed with 50 per cent oxygen, so doesn't have the same effect as pure nitrogen and can give you brain damage if taken incorrectly.

We just accept verbal abuse as a run-of-the-mill occurrence. Certainly, most of it goes unreported. It tends to be linked to drugs and alcohol, and people can be almost intolerable when they've had too much to drink. I've never understood it, because when I have a drink, I turn into a lover rather than a fighter. But it turns some people into maniacs. And it's not just that they become aggressive, they also become non-compliant. You'll ask them to sit down and they'll stand up. You'll ask them to stand up and they'll lie down. You'll ask them to be quiet and they'll start shouting in your face. Should we accept it? No. Do we? Yes, because we don't have a choice.

I think some people speak to and treat us like rubbish simply because we're wearing a uniform, which dehumanises us. What they don't seem to understand is that, despite the uniform, we're real people with real feelings. And some of the abuse is down to an ingrained hatred of authority. These people see us as part of the establishment, and therefore the enemy. They are unable to distinguish between us and the police. But we're not there to ask difficult questions or arrest anyone, we're there to hopefully save a life, or at the very least help someone.

I should stress that the vast majority of people are nice and understanding. But there is enough disrespect for it to become very wearing. The voices and blows of the abusive are so loud and concussive that they sometimes drown out everything else. Someone being nasty can make me feel so low and despairing of humanity, especially if all you're trying to do is help them. And in practical terms, the verbal, physical and sexual assaults are putting yet more strain on the ambulance service. A fifth of the ambulance workers polled by the GMB took sick leave after an attack and 37 per cent said they had considered quitting the job because of the threat of violence.

People will stick notes on the ambulance's windscreen: 'DO NOT PARK ACROSS MY DRIVE AGAIN!' I read them and think, *Sorry, mate, but your neighbour has just had a cardiac arrest*. We honestly do the best we can not to park like idiots and inconvenience anyone. It's not as if we turn up to a job and say, 'Tell you what, Dave, reverse a couple of feet so that BMW can't get out,' but we have to park as close as possible to the scene. An ambulance is even bigger than it looks because it has a tail lift, and we also need room to manoeuvre a stretcher. So there's more to it than just parking up, and when there's a lack of space, we sometimes end up blocking one or more cars in.

What people don't seem to realise is that leaving nasty notes can get you nicked. In 2018, a woman in Stoke was fined £120 for leaving a note on an ambulance, demanding it be moved, despite the fact it had been sent to her next-door neighbour who was having breathing difficulties. To her credit, she had a beautiful way with words: 'I couldn't give a shit if the whole street collasped [*sic*]. Now move your van from outside my house.' What a charmer.

I once turned up at a block of flats for an elderly lady with chest pains. It sounded like she might have a problem with her heart, so I returned to the ambulance to grab the wheelchair and lower the tail lift. I went back to collect the patient and, while I was bringing her out, a woman started banging on her car horn and screaming at us: 'You can't park it there, you dickheads! I've got places to be! Shift the fucking ambulance now or I'll fucking kill you both!' As I said, these people tend to have a wonderful way with words. The poor woman in the wheelchair didn't have a clue what was happening. For an easy life, I wheeled her back inside while my partner moved the ambulance to let this other woman out.

I find it impossible to understand the mentality of people like that. In that particular case, it wasn't just a lack of love for her fellow humans, it was lack of love for the woman who lived next door and had fallen ill. We phoned the police, gave them her car registration and they gave her a ticking off. That's all we could do, because you can't afford to snap in situations like that. They can call you every name under the sun, but if you tell them where to go, you're just adding fuel to the fire. Besides, we had a patient to look after and arguing the toss over a parking space isn't really a priority.

Only the other day, we received an email telling us that a complaint had been made about an ambulance driving on the wrong side of the road. To be fair, the sender of the email did suggest the complaint had no merit. But they still felt the need to tell us to drive carefully, despite the fact we're trained to drive on the wrong side of the road. Where else do you want us to drive when there are massive traffic jams and we're trying to reach a critically ill patient?

Most of our fellow road users know the drill when they see and hear an ambulance. I assume some of the problems we have on the road are down to a lack of awareness among new drivers. Although I think others simply have difficulty understanding that the 5-ton vehicle coming up behind them, painted yellow and with a screaming siren and flashing blue lights, isn't doing all that just to show off, it's on its way to help someone in need. I'll be driving along, five cars will yield, but the car directly in front of me will speed up and overtake the cars that have pulled over. Do they really think those cars have pulled over especially for them? Or do they just see it as an opportunity to get home that much quicker? Then there are those who think it's fun to follow in our slipstream, as if we're bombing round Silverstone. I honestly don't know what goes on in these people's heads.

The lack of respect for staff in A&E never ceases to amaze me and I have no idea where it came from. I've witnessed terrible abuse aimed at doctors and nurses – 'I've been waiting here for hours, you fuckin' bitch!' – although I've never seen a physical attack, probably because hospital security is pretty good and there are usually quite a few coppers milling about, having brought injured suspects in for assessment before taking them to the station.

Whenever I see someone mouthing off in A&E, I'm reminded of that episode of *Only Fools and Horses,* in which Del Boy punches a drunk bloke who is being abusive in the hospital. That's exactly how people behave, and I'm not surprised the studio audience gave Del Boy a round of applause (if I remember rightly, one of Del Boy's next lines was, 'I bet you wish you'd gone private,' which was bang on as well).

In real life, Del Boy probably would have been arrested and the drunk walked away scot-free. I had a colleague who was former army and had served in the Middle East. He was great at his job and one of the good guys, just a lovely bloke. One night, somebody flicked a cigarette at his partner. In the military, you're trained to look after the man on either side of you. So he followed this idiot into the hospital and dragged him out by the scruff of his neck. He didn't hit him, he just deposited him outside. But as night follows day, he got suspended. This is a military hero, who put his life on the line for the country. And for that, he'll always be a hero to me, whatever happens next.

Older people tend to be more respectful. They under-stand what a fantastic service the NHS provides and tend to be very stoic. But that love has slowly been eroded. I'm not about to start bashing millennials, but a lot of younger people don't see the NHS as a marvel to be thankful for, they see it as an entitlement. People break a finger, march into A&E and want it seen to immediately. And when they are told they will have to join a queue, because there are other patients who are critically unwell, they take it as a personal affront. There will be old people sitting there with broken hips and pelvises, not saying a word, while a young mum is kicking off because her child, who has grazed his knee, has been waiting fifteen minutes.

———

Town centre, Sunday morning, about 1 a.m. A girl in her mid-twenties is in a heap on the floor, her foot facing the wrong way. We jump out of the ambulance, introduce ourselves and advise her that she really needs to go to hospital to get her ankle seen to. Somewhat surprisingly, she tells us to leave her alone, or words to that effect. When we tell her that we're only trying to help her and that if she doesn't come with us she might lose her foot, she starts screaming, 'Stop touching me!'

Now we're a bit spooked. I request a female crew but there aren't any. Eventually, and after soaking up ten more minutes of dog's abuse, we flag down a passing police car. They try their best to get her to see sense, and she tells them to sling their hook as well. Eventually, I assume because the alcohol is starting to wear off and the pain is kicking in, she agrees to get in the ambulance. But she's still not happy about it.

We wheel her into A&E and she's shouting and screaming about how horrible we've been to her. The head sister comes to see what all the commotion is about and the girl barks at her, 'When are you going to see me? I want to be seen now! I want to go home!' This girl is one of the vilest people I've ever dealt with – think Veruca Salt from *Charlie and the Chocolate Factory*, except after ten bottles of Blue WKD – but the ability of A&E staff to let this kind of abuse just slide off their backs is nothing short of miraculous. Later, I discover that she's a primary school teacher. I'm confident she doesn't behave like that in her classroom, so I'm not sure why she thinks it's acceptable to behave like that in my place of work.

Wonderfully, the head sister sent the teacher a letter, something along the lines of: 'You attended our A&E department on Sunday morning and I was disgusted with the way you spoke to my staff and the ambulance staff who brought you in. I suggest you review the way you behaved and send a letter of apology to the people you insulted.' I thought it was absolutely brilliant that the sister had done that, not least because it was the kind of thing a teacher would say to a disobedient pupil. The teacher never sent an apology.

However, for the sake of balance, I should point out

that older people don't always get it right. I've been to a lot of jobs in bingo halls – for the obvious reason that a lot of old people play bingo. On one occasion, me and my partner were attending to a lady who had become unwell and people were shushing us and telling us to be quiet. One of my colleagues attended a cardiac arrest in the local Mecca and, while he was doing CPR, the caller carried on reading out the numbers. It was like a scene from *Phoenix Nights*: 'Never been kissed, one and six. And could the lads attending to the stroke victim kindly keep the noise down ...'

———

We're called back to the guy who punched me in his flat. Alas, he's a regular caller. We knock, he opens the door and says, 'Piss off!' before slamming the door in our faces. We knock again, he opens the door and I say, 'You phoned for us, mate.' He replies, 'Stop molestering me! Leave me alone!' before slamming the door closed again. Knock. Knock. This time when he opens the door, he's holding his phone above his head and clicking away, as if he's taking pictures of us. Every time he clicks the button, he shouts, 'Evidence!' But it's one of those old Nokia phones with no camera. David Bailey impression over, he slams the door closed again, and we can hear him on his phone: 'Police? I've just been raped by two ambulancemen ...' Not ideal.

For whatever reason, mental illness has gone through the roof. I'd go as far as to say it's a pandemic. I see an awful lot of mentally ill people living on the streets or on their own without much support and unable to cope with the daily stresses of life. It's not unusual for me to spend a large chunk of a shift dealing with mentally ill patients. They're often people at the end of their tether, who have cut their wrists or taken an overdose. It's humbling to be the first port of call for people such as this and hopefully be able to help them take the first step on the road to recovery. And I can often draw on my own experiences to help understand their predicament. But we don't get an awful lot of training in how to treat mentally ill patients, including what or what not to say.

———

I've taken people into hospital who have been sectioned or were feeling suicidal, returned two days later and bumped into them again. I've said to them, 'How come you're back?' And they replied, 'I've not left.' They're essentially living in a medical hospital, waiting for a mental health bed to become available. It's not uncommon for people to go to their GP and get a referral to a mental health professional, only for it to take three or four months. The GP might give them some pills, but they're not going to cure you, they're only going to mask the symptoms. And, once again, it's the ambulance service that picks up the pieces, when people waiting for an assessment, desperate for support and guidance and crying out for help, harm themselves. Whatever is wrong with someone, we do everything we can. But sometimes it's just not enough.

12

THE SEEMINGLY HUMDRUM

Even an ambulance person's everyday jobs can be deeply unsettling. When you're trained how to do CPR, your patient is a dummy. Dummies don't have emotions, or eyes that stare straight into yours, or friends telling you what to do. Dummies don't foam or vomit, they don't have ribs that break or cardiac arrests in tiny bathrooms. When you're doing CPR for real, the patient won't be presented on a nice flat bed, at exactly the right height. He or she might be curled up in a toilet cubicle or face down under a pier on a beach.

Name a place and the chances are I've done CPR there, or know someone who has. And when you start pounding on their chest, you will be able to feel and hear their ribs popping, crunching and cracking, as if they're nothing more than twigs. Some elderly people have a DNAR order in place, but many don't. That means we don't have a choice but to do CPR on them, which is highly unlikely to work. It's the law, but is it morally right? Either way, it's not nice for whoever has to do it.

I should make clear that I don't describe jobs in such graphic detail for reasons of gratuitousness or vicarious voyeurism, but to impress upon the reader the stark realities of an ambulance person's existence. Because if the reader doesn't understand the stark realities of an ambulance person's existence, they will never begin to understand what happened to me.

Before I started working out on the road as a technician, I received nothing at all in terms of psychological training. No old sweats came in and described what they'd seen and what we should expect. Nobody took us to the morgue to view dead bodies. Nobody told us that we'd probably see decapitated bodies at traffic accidents, people swinging from ropes in lofts, dead babies and screaming relatives. And I didn't ask. It's not as if I didn't want to get a reputa-tion as someone who asks difficult questions – or, in other words, a trouble-maker – I didn't even think it was odd. And had I asked, 'What are the possible mental effects of what I'm about to do?' I'm pretty sure someone would have said, 'What you on about, son? Just watch and learn.'

After seeing my first dead body on the job, my colleague

said to me, 'Are you okay? Because you'll see this a lot.' What if I wasn't? Tough, get on with it. Those in charge would no doubt argue that nothing can prepare an ambulance person for the things they'll see. As I've already illustrated, in some ways they're right. But I think more of an effort needs to be made.

Every ambulance person has their kryptonite, and mine is bones sticking out of bodies. I see a fair few bones pointing where they shouldn't be on football and rugby pitches on Saturday and Sunday mornings. I went to a rugby match once and this bloke's shin bone was sticking out at a right angle, piercing the skin. Its brilliant whiteness amazed me. But once I'd stopped appreciating its strange beauty, all I could think was, *Oh. My. God. What the hell are we gonna do here?*

First thing, pain relief – although we were never going to be able to relieve the pain completely. We wrapped a vacuum splint around the joint, placed the patient on the trolley, made sure he was as comfortable as possible and ferried him to hospital, where hopefully the surgeons put him on the road to recovery.

Another time, I went to a little girl who had been hit by a car after getting off the school bus and running into the road. She told me her leg hurt, but I couldn't work out what the problem was. I didn't want to be cutting her clothes off in the middle of the street, so I said to her, 'You know what I'll do? I'll carry you to the ambulance so that we can get away from all these people watching.' When I picked the girl up, I looked down and saw that her thigh was snapped in two and hanging limp. When I lifted it back up, she started screaming, which made me think that I shouldn't have moved her. In the ambulance game we call that 'continuing professional development', which means learning from mistakes.

I also attended a guy who had slipped over getting out of the shower. His leg was broken so badly and at such a strange angle that we couldn't get him down the stairs without banging it against the bannisters. You become good at problem-solving in the ambulance service, what with all the moving and handling we do. But this poor chap was more precious than an odd-shaped piece of furniture. So we had no choice but to call the fire service, who removed an upstairs window and brought him down in a cherry picker.

Another time, we were sent to an 18-year-old lad who was described as generally unwell, vomiting and suffering with a high temperature. On the way there, I thought it would be another patient with a bit of man flu. But when we turned up, this lad was yellow, so that he looked like one of the Simpsons, and clearly had some organ failure going on. We got him into the ambulance, gave him some fluids through a drip and raced him off to the hospital.

The doctors diagnosed something called leptospirosis (or Weil's disease), which is an infection spread in the urine of animals. This lad had been working in a pub cellar changing barrels and presumably caught the infection from rat wee. He nearly died, just from biting his nails, and was in intensive care for a month. And his poor mum and dad had been telling him to sleep it off. They weren't to know what was wrong with him, and it's not something ambulance people are trained to spot either. The lad made a full recovery, but it was a close shave.

And it's not just the dramatic stuff that can make a dent in an ambulance person's armour. The seemingly humdrum can drip, drip, drip and act like water wearing down a stone. If the public knew about everything that happened out there, they'd be horrified. If journalists reported everything that happened in a 24-hour period, the local paper would be like a copy of the *Yellow Pages*. So many of the patients I've treated were just going about their daily lives and – BOOM – everything changed in an instant. A bit of water on a bathroom floor, some spilt soup in a kitchen, a slight lapse of concentration while driving, and suddenly I'm looking down on them or peering at them through a mangled car door. And, at that moment, I'm the only face they want to see. My job gives me a very acute appreciation of the fragility of life. Including mine.

In the ambulance service, one small slip can cause months of almost unbearable stress. Needle-stick or sharps injuries are the bane of anyone who works in healthcare. If you accidentally prick yourself with a needle when treating a patient, you can be at risk of HIV, hepatitis B and C and all sorts of other nasty stuff. Needle-stick injuries are often the result of carelessness but can also happen if a patient is being a bit combative or thrashing about. If you do suffer a needle-stick injury, occupational health will put you on hardcore anti-viral medication called PEP (post-exposure prophylaxis), which can have severe side-effects, including diarrhoea, headaches, nausea, vomiting and fatigue. But worse than that is the months of waiting to be given the all-clear.

I've never suffered a needle-stick injury (touch wood), but I was once doing CPR on a guy in cardiac arrest, went to open his airwave and he spewed blood all over my face. Occupational health asked if I washed my face straightaway, to which I replied I didn't, because I was busy trying to save this guy's life. He was ninety years old, so occupational health classed him as low risk (high risk patients are usually drug users). My problem was that the patient died, so they couldn't get his permission to take a blood sample. They didn't put me on PEP, but I had to go on a six-month watch list, which involved regular blood tests. I wasn't overly stressed, and I was eventually given the all-clear, but it gave me an insight into how horrible it must be for those colleagues who have suffered a needle-stick injury while treating someone with HIV or hepatitis C.

On any given day, I might fail to resuscitate an elderly man who's had a cardiac arrest, successfully treat a fitting child and tell someone that their mum has died. I couldn't tell you how many people I've seen dead on a toilet. It wasn't just Elvis Presley who breathed his last on the throne. It's so common, we call it the 'death poo'. We went to one woman in a care home who died mid-evacuation. At least I think she did, I didn't check. The family were on their way, so me and my partner grabbed an arm and a leg each, lugged the woman over to the bed, put her under the bedclothes and tucked her in, so that when her family arrived, she looked nice and peaceful. We also tidied the room up, swept the floor and straightened her hair. I've picked up so many tips like this during my years on the job, little things that make a horrible situation a little more tolerable. Obviously, we had to tell her family that she'd passed away in the toilet, but they didn't need to see that.

However, while it's part of our job to make a loved one's death easier to deal with, we don't get to choose what we do and don't see.

I once turned up to someone who had died in front of a fire. Imagine a slow-cooked piece of pork and you're in the right area. I went to another lady who had been dead for over a week. When we tried to roll her over, half her face remained stuck to the carpet. I've crept through a graveyard in the middle of the night, trying to find someone who was suicidal. He'd sat down next to his mum's grave, popped a load of pills and called us. Unfortunately, we didn't know where his mum's plot was. While we were looking, plastic windmills on gravestones whistled in the wind. I don't know what was spookier, the sound of those windmills or the uncontrollable sobbing of the patient, somewhere in the darkness. I've driven an ambulance around a park for half an hour, trying to locate a patient with chest pains. When we finally found our man, slumped on a bench, I jumped on top of him and gave him CPR, only for him to die on me.

People often think heart attacks and cardiac arrests are the same, but they're not. Symptoms of a heart attack (otherwise known as a myocardial infarction, or MI) include tightness or aching in the chest, which might spread to the neck, jaw or back; nausea, indigestion, heartburn or abdominal pain; shortness of breath; cold sweats; fatigue and dizziness. But someone can have a heart attack and not even know it. And these days, if you're having a heart attack and it's dealt with in good time, the survival rate is quite high. When we turn up, we'll do an ECG and if the patient is having a heart attack, we take them into a specialist heart centre. After the surgeons have done a

PPCI (primary percutaneous coronary intervention, or angioplasty, which is a procedure used to treat the narrowed coronary arteries of the heart), the patient might be back home in a couple of days.

A cardiac arrest is when a patient's heart suddenly stops pumping blood around the body, which means their brain gets starved of oxygen. As a result, there are no symptoms. And once someone has had a cardiac arrest, there is only about a 10 per cent chance of survival. That surprises a lot of people, probably because they've watched a lot of medical dramas on TV, in which people are regularly brought back from the brink with CPR. At the same time, most of the people I've managed to save were the beneficiaries of good quality CPR before we arrived on the scene.

One time, we were called to a guy who had collapsed on a treadmill in a gym. The gym staff did their bit before we turned up and gave him a whack of the old defib. By the time we arrived at A&E, he was sat up talking. But that was one of the few occasions I've seen someone survive a cardiac arrest outside of hospital. There have been other times I've turned up to a patient who has already received CPR and seems right as rain. Of course, they might not have had a cardiac arrest in the first place, although that's just me being cynical.

Teaching CPR is easy enough and if everyone knew how to do it, it would save lives. We saw that recently, when the former footballer and England manager Glenn Hoddle had a cardiac arrest in a studio and a sound engineer who knew CPR kept him alive until an ambulance arrived. They're talking about teaching it in schools, which would be the right thing to do. It would take ten minutes during morning assembly. That said, while it's easy enough to teach how to spot when someone has had a cardiac arrest – usually it's a case of bang, they're suddenly on the floor – and administering it is pretty simple (no mouth to mouth any more, just hard and fast pressing on the centre of the chest, like Vinnie Jones says on the advert), you're only supposed to administer CPR when someone's not breathing or their heart's not beating. And teaching people how to feel for a pulse is more difficult.

Even we get confused sometimes. I turned up at one job in a working men's club to find a motorcycle paramedic already on the scene. This lad was doing CPR and every time he pounded on the patient's chest, his arms started rising up, as if he was trying to push the paramedic off. I didn't know the paramedic very well, but I knew this wasn't supposed to happen. So I said to him, 'Mate, what are you doing?' And he replied, 'I've got no idea what's going on here, but as soon as I stop, his heart stops as well.' So I let him get on with it. I looked it up afterwards and discovered it's called CPR induced consciousness. The CPR the guy was administering was so good, every time he pounded on the patient's chest, it was getting the circulation to his head.

Very occasionally, a member of the public knows too much. Or thinks they do. I turned up at one job to find a woman performing CPR on a patient. When we asked her to step aside, she replied, 'It's okay, I'm a veterinary nurse.' What did she expect us to say? 'Oh, I didn't realise. We'll leave it with you . . .' To be fair, she probably knew what she was doing, because most mammals are similar once you cut them open. But can you imagine if a dog keeled over, I happened to be on the scene and a veterinary nurse turned up? 'As you were, these poodles aren't much different to humans . . .'

I've given patients CPR while a husband has stood over me shouting: 'Why are you still here? Why haven't you taken her to hospital? Help her!' It's part of my job to explain that I'm doing what I'm doing to give their loved one the best chance of survival, because it's so difficult to administer good CPR in a moving ambulance (although new CPR machines are being rolled out across the country, which allow us to get on with the other jobs we need to do during a resuscitation attempt).

People respond to trauma in lots of different ways. I can tell one person they're having a heart attack (which is a strange thing to have to tell someone, and a big responsibility) and they'll be completely unfazed: 'Oh, okay.

So what now?' I told one guy he was probably having a heart attack and he replied, 'Erm, the problem is, it's my wedding day. I'm supposed to be getting married in three hours . . .' Obviously, we still had to take him into hospital and I can only assume his big day was cancelled. I hope his bride-to-be understood. I'm sure some people suspect they've had a heart attack and don't even report it, because they're afraid of hospitals or simply too busy.

Another person will be terrified (as I would be) and shaking like a leaf. So it's my job to try to keep a lid on things. We don't just burst into someone's living room, do our assessments, suddenly announce the patient is having a heart attack and bundle them into the ambulance. The last thing you want when someone is having a heart attack is to get their heart racing. Instead, we'll say something like, 'The ECG suggests you're having a heart attack. The good news is, the medical world has come a long way. We'll take you direct to a specialist healthcare facility, where they'll hopefully be able to rectify the problem.' We don't hang about, but we calmly explain what the hospital procedure will involve: 'Don't worry, it's nothing major. They'll go straight into a vein, normally one in your wrist or your leg, pop a couple of tubes in to keep the artery from becoming blocked again and hopefully you'll be out in a couple of days.' We can usually see the relief on the patient's face. They realise they're in kind hands and they're going to get the best treatment possible.

There's no real good way of delivering bad news, but there are better ways than others. Ambulance people can't administer sedative drugs, so we use words as sedatives instead. As Frank Carson used to say, it's the way you tell 'em.

13

RIGHT PLACE, RIGHT TIME

I might think I'm on my way to a routine job and then something else comes up that we need to attend instead. I suppose it's being in the right place at the right time. Once, I was driving to the hospital when I saw a little girl of about three pushing a toy pram down the street. My first reaction was, 'Aah, look at that little girl with the pram.' But then I realised she had no shoes on and there were no adults with her. I pulled over, asked her where her mummy and daddy were, where she lived and where she was going. She didn't know the answer to any of my questions. We didn't know what to do with her, so we called the police. They had a report of a missing child and managed to reunite the girl with her parents at the hospital. I assume social services had a look at that one, because if we hadn't driven past, anything could have happened to her.

Two colleagues of mine were once flagged down by a woman in the process of giving birth in her car. She'd driven to hospital and the baby had started emerging while she was in the car park of the maternity department. That's a tough enough job as it is, but try doing it when the mum is sat in the driver's seat of a Fiat Panda. Personally, I would have run and got a midwife, but these two lads got stuck in and delivered the baby with no hitches. I've also heard stories about babies being delivered in lay-bys, a post office, the car park of a Chinese restaurant and on the pavement outside Primark.

Sometimes, though, something comes out of the blue and takes the wind out of me. We're halfway through a shift and on our way to a headache. To be fair, there are such things as thunderclap headaches, which are apparently agonising. Or a headache might be a bleed on the brain and therefore life-threatening. But usually they're just headaches. Trundling along the motorway, we pass a moped. Its exhaust falls off, gets caught on the wheel and the woman riding on the back somersaults through the air and lands on her face. The headache is on ice.

Jobs on motorways are some of the hairiest we can do. Whenever I'm called to one, I always hope the police have arrived before us, so that they've already closed the road.

Once, I beat them to a rollover and turned up to find a car upside down in the middle lane. People have their own business to attend to and only care about getting through before the motorway gets closed, so even after we've parked in the so-called fend-off position – diagonally across the road so that we block off two lanes – cars will try to squeeze past us. They might be on their way to see a dying relative. But probably not.

On this occasion, cars pull over to let us through, we put the blue lights on, park up, put on our high-vis jackets and grab everything from the back (we're not allowed to go back in case someone crashes into us). My mate jumps out of the ambulance while I call the control room to tell them we're going to have to bin off the other job and ask them to send the police. Meanwhile, my mate is shouting at me to come quick. I can tell straightaway that this woman has done herself some serious mischief. She's wearing one of those helmets that only covers the head and not the face, which is a bloody mess. Worse, she isn't breathing. We immediately start CPR and all I can hear in the background is the rider of the moped, who I assume is her partner, shouting, 'No! No! No!'

We put the patient on a stretcher, get her into the ambulance and manage to get her heart beating, although we still have to assist her breathing. I can tell just by looking at her that her injuries are too significant for her to survive.

Ambulance people become very good at knowing if someone is beyond help. White people go grey. It's more difficult to tell with black people, for the simple reason that they have darker skin. But people who are critically unwell often get a sense of impending doom, which is reflected in the expression on their faces. It's a ghastly look of fear, that their life is slipping away and they've got nothing left to fight it. They won't be able to speak, but their eyes will say to you, 'I'm dying here, aren't I?' I wonder what someone thinks, when they know their time on earth is about to be up?

We rush the woman to hospital, from where we take her to a major trauma centre. About twelve hours later, the woman dies in the intensive care unit. It isn't the outcome we wanted, but there are positives we can take from it. Had we not been driving past when the accident happened, there is every chance she would have died on the side of the road. But we were able to give her and her family the gift of time and the chance to say goodbye. Second to saving somebody's life, that's the best thing an ambulance person can do.

———

It's the kind of cold winter's day that makes you want to be tucked up snug and warm under your duvet. There is a big cycle ride taking place in the evening, which is lovely, but also means inevitable crashes and having to nose our ambulance through forests of bikes. We're on our way to one of these stricken cyclists when we see a load of people gathered by the sea wall, roaring and screaming. I wind down the window and someone starts shouting at us, 'There's a man in the water! There's a man in the water!'

People see an ambulance person and assume they can do everything – apprehend criminals, rescue cats from trees, perform open heart surgery. But my first thought is, *I'm definitely not David Hasselhoff.* I contact the coastguard, but the rescue officers have to get to the boathouse and launch, which means an arrival time of ten minutes at best.

The sea is rough and there are waves crashing over the wall. Apparently, this homeless guy had been walking his dog, the dog had jumped in the sea and its owner had jumped in after it. We trot over, have a look over the top of the wall and see this guy struggling to keep his head above water, while being repeatedly smashed against the steps and sucked back out again. Every now and again his head disappears, before popping back up. We quickly realise that this bloke doesn't have ten minutes. As for the dog, he's sitting next to us drip-drying, having jumped out pretty soon after jumping in. His calm exterior and the contented expression on his face suggests he really couldn't care less.

I can't help thinking of a story I once heard: a dog

jumped in the sea, its owner tried to save him, a policeman tried to save the owner and all three ended up dead. But we have to try something. My partner grabs a life ring attached to a rope and tries to land it over the guy's head. He tries it once, he tries it again, but even when he lands it close, the sea is so choppy that within a couple of seconds the ring is about 10 metres away. And then – bingo! – my mate lands the ring over the flailing man and we manage to reel him in. The man doesn't have a good enough hold on the ring that we can drag him out, so we run down the steps, I grab hold of my mate's legs, he leans over the side and hauls this guy out, as if he's a gigantic fish we've landed.

Everyone is cheering and telling us well done, but we don't really have time for any photos with our catch. In fact, our work has barely started, because this guy is now in cardiac arrest. We have to carry him up about thirty steps and we don't have any gear with us, because we've left it in the ambulance. We get him in the back of the ambulance, do a round of CPR, and what happens next is like something from the movies: he suddenly coughs and water spurts from his mouth. He's back in the room, which hardly ever happens. Seconds later, there is a knock on the window: it's the coastguard.

'Everything all right?'

'Stand down, pal, we don't need you any more . . .'

We rush the guy into hospital and he lives to tell the tale.

We'd gone above and beyond the call of duty, to the extent that we thought we were going to get a roasting from management. We didn't overcommit, although one or both of us could quite easily have gone in. And I don't think anyone in our position would have stood back and watched the guy drown. But sometimes in the ambulance service, we are faced with situations where we don't have a choice but to breach health and safety guidelines in order to save someone.

Unbeknown to us, an off-duty police chief inspector had been watching us pull this bloke out of the drink, while trying to hold the crowd back. He sent a letter of commendation to our bosses and we ended up getting a couple of bravery awards. I'm not sure how brave it was really. There is this theory that the more people who are around when someone needs saving, the less likely anyone is to help, because they all expect someone else to act first. But if you're the only person on the scene, you will do something. In the case of the drowning man, we were the only people with blue flashing lights and wearing a uniform, so everyone expected us to do the business.

The irony of being in the right place at the right time is that it's a result of the patient being in the wrong place at the wrong time. A colleague once drove past a woman with a head injury: it turned out a sign had blown off a shop and fallen on her. My colleague couldn't save her life, but he could make sure she was given every possible chance.

I'm driving along with a patient in the back one day, and a guy flags us down outside a building site. I shout to my partner in the back, 'I don't know what's going on, but someone needs our help.' Fortunately, there is a carer with our current patient in the back of the ambulance, so we decide to investigate. It's not ideal, but sometimes we just have to spin two plates at once. There is a plaster wall around the building site to keep the public out, but through a little opening I can see a guy laid out on a cherry picker. I grab my mate, get a kindly member of the public to give me a leg-up over the wall and my partner chucks all our gear over. Someone jumps on the cherry picker and lowers it to the ground, and it transpires that a big bolt has come loose and fallen on this guy's head, smashing his hard hat to pieces.

We try to establish what we call neutral alignment of the neck, to protect it while assessing the man's airway (quite tricky on a cherry picker), which means my hands are cradling the back of this guy's head. It feels like mashed potato, or a cracked boiled egg. Where once there was a skull, there is now shards of bone intermingled with soft tissue. We can't really leave our other patient in the back of the ambulance, but luckily another ambulance turns up and takes him. By this time, I'm covered in blood up to my elbows. A helicopter lands and flies the patient to a trauma centre. I've got no idea whether he survived or not.

Another day, another building site, another nightmare from start to finish. A brickie was building a second-floor wall and, for whatever reason, the wall toppled over on top of him, breaking his legs. There are still no stairs in the building, so technically, as far as our health and safety people are concerned, we shouldn't go up there, because that would mean we're working at heights. But how are we going to get this bloke down if we don't?

We have something called HARTs (Hazardous Area Response Teams), who are like the SAS of the ambulance service. At pretty much every major incident, a HART is on the scene. They would have been in the thick of it at the Manchester bombing and the Salisbury chemical attack, and are also straight in whenever there is a large-scale road traffic accident, a train crash, a collapsed building or a big fire (although they sometimes find themselves extracting bariatric patients, which I can't imagine they're thrilled about).

Us common or garden ambulance people are a bit envious of them, because HARTs have the shiniest vehicles, the smartest uniforms, lots of James Bond kit (all-terrain vehicles, flotation devices for working on water, special ladders, breathing apparatus). Members of HARTs are even equipped with body armour, so that they can work at terrorist incidents, when a bomber or shooter is still at large.

One night, an address came on the screen and just as we pulled up, someone came on our radio and told us to hang back, because there was reason to believe there was a bomb inside the house. How do you react to that? 'Oh. Thanks for letting us know . . .'

I reversed a few hundred yards down the road, the cops turned up and informed us that they believed the chap inside the house had been making pipe bombs. He wasn't a terrorist, he was just a pipe bomb hobbyist. Who knew? They told us to rendezvous at the police station car park and await further instruction. I assume we were on standby in case a bomb went off, although no one told us.

The HART arrived, which is when we knew how seriously the police were taking it. As well as all their James Bond kit, HARTs turn up with a portable control unit, from which they run the operation. But we refer to it as a brew wagon, because it has a kettle in it and we always fill our boots. Hot on the heels of the HART, a bomb disposal team turns up and a police sergeant says to us, 'Right, we're gonna have to evacuate the car park. When we arrested the suspect earlier today, we confiscated a rucksack, which is now in the police station.' As we were leaving, the bomb disposal team were disappearing inside the police station.

It was like a Keystone Cops film. The bomb disposal team did its thing, we got a couple of cuppas out of the job and I assume the bomb maker got nicked and banged up. If you will have strange hobbies . . .

Alas, in the case of the man under a wall on a building site, a Chinook doesn't appear, dispensing members of a HART on ropes. So we grab a ladder, climb up it and attend to the patient. We've now crossed a red line, because if we fall off and do ourselves a mischief, we'll be told it's our fault – 'What are you doing climbing up ladders? Have you done the course?' We call the fire service to get the man down, and off we toddle to the hospital.

Even when an ambulance person isn't in uniform, the instinct to help will kick in if we think someone is in peril. One day, I was wandering back from the shop when I heard what sounded like a smoke alarm coming from the sheltered accommodation across the road. It's common to hear alarms going off and for it to mean nothing. But, being a nosey git, I went and had a look. I tracked the alarm down to a second floor flat, pushed the door open and was met with thick smoke and a burning armchair. It turned out that this old girl had fallen asleep with a ciggie in her hand.

But while I was trying to usher her out, all she was bothered about was finding her cat: 'I can't leave! I've got to save Felix!' Some old people become so set in their ways that they have little appreciation of danger or their own vulnerability. I was coughing and spluttering, even though my T-shirt was covering my face, and by the time I got this woman out – minus her cat – she was covered head to toe in soot. While I was waiting for the fire brigade to turn up, I went around knocking on doors and telling people to get out. The fire brigade extinguished the flaming armchair in seconds, but I never found out what happened to the cat.

I was driving home from a late shift when I happened to look up and see someone sat on a bridge over a motorway. I went around the roundabout again, just to make sure I'd seen correctly, and sure enough there was a young woman sitting on the wrong side of the railings, with her legs dangling over the edge. I phoned the police (which I was a bit nervous about, because my MOT had expired that morning) and thought I'd better go and persuade this woman that jumping was a bad idea. Or at least try to.

I parked the car up, hopped out and said, 'My name's Dan, I work for the ambulance service. I was on my way home when I saw you. What's happening?'

She replied, 'I'm just waiting for a lorry to be honest with you.'

This was a bit of a conundrum. Should I start talking about why she was thinking about jumping off a bridge? Or would it be a bad idea to dredge all that stuff up? Should I try to grab her and pull her to safety? What if I tried and she fell? I was a bit out of my depth. In the end I plumped for, 'Do you want to come and sit in my car and get warm? I've left the engine running.'

I saw a police car go flying past and wondered why it hadn't stopped, before realising that they were off to close the motorway. Eventually, a lovely copper called Macca turned up, who was on the scene when I got punched in the flat. Macca was the nicest guy you could ever meet, a proper old-school bobby, who happened to have cancer. He should have been tucked up in bed, but was still desperate to help people in need. Between us, we managed to talk her out of jumping and get her back over the railings. And when an ambulance turned up, she was detained under Section 136 of the Mental Health Act – as a patient, not a law-breaker – and taken to hospital. On the drive home, all I could think was, *What if I'd stopped for a chat after work? If I had driven past five minutes later, would that lorry have turned up?* As it is, I hope the woman got the help she needed and managed to turn her life around.

On the odd occasion, we'll be in the right place at the wrong time for a member of the public. Me and Paul were winding our way down a country lane one evening, on our way back to the station for a rare dinner break, when we came across a car crashed into a bush on quite a severe bend. Bang went the dinner break. The two lads were fine and told us a mate was on his way to pull them out. So I said, 'That's fine, but we can't stay here for ever. We have to phone the police so that they can seal off the scene.' One of the blokes went into a panic and started telling us not to phone the Old Bill. And when I assured him it wasn't a problem and that the police would just mop things up before the recovery came, this bloke took off across a field. His mate was shouting after him, calling him every name under the sun.

The bloke who stayed behind wouldn't have been much good under interrogation, because within seconds he'd told us that he was the owner of the car but his mate was driving, while pissed and without insurance. So when the police arrived, a couple of them went straight after him. Me and Paul were talking to the copper who had remained on the scene when I suddenly got a strong whiff of gas. When I looked under the crashed car – which was still running – I saw it had taken out a gas main. We jumped back into the ambulance, blocked one end of the road, the police blocked the other end and we called the fire brigade, only to be told it wasn't their job and that we should get on to the gas board instead. The leaking gas main backed on to a caravan park, so I had to go knocking on caravan doors and suggest the occupants made themselves scarce.

An hour or so later, someone from the gas board turned up and slapped what looked like a big blob of Play-Doh over the top of the main. So while we missed out on dinner at the station that day, maybe we stopped a few caravans from being blown up. Not really my job, but I was happy to do it.

We ambulance people often find ourselves performing to a crowd, often with people filming us. Even if we're trying to save someone who's choking. Whenever we get called to a choking, it's uncommon for the person to still need our help when we arrive. It's usually a partial airway obstruction, and whatever it was they had in their throat – a fish bone, a piece of bread – has been dislodged. Thankfully, I've only ever been called to one child choking (they normally stick things up their noses or in their ears) but by the time we rocked up to the nursery, a member of staff had removed the offending item, in this case a humble grape. But on the few occasions I've been called to full airway obstructions, we've arrived too late to be able to save them.

One Sunday afternoon, we get a call to a carvery restaurant. Our screen simply said: MALE CHOKING. We're only around the corner from the restaurant, so arrive in a couple of minutes. As we pull into the car park, someone is frantically waving at us outside. And when we swing the doors open, the waft of carvery – old, sweaty vegetables and cheap lager – almost knocks us backwards.

If you've ever been to a carvery on a Sunday afternoon, you'll know exactly how busy this place was. And the prospect of missing out on a giant Yorkshire pudding from the buffet is apparently far more worrying than the man lying on his back in the middle of the restaurant, turning blue. Wading through overly enthusiastic diners, carrying plates piled up to the ceiling, I can't help thinking, *You're never gonna eat all that!*

As anyone who has been on a first aid course will know, this is a case of ABC – Airway, Breathing, Circulation. So the first thing I do is have a look down his throat, where I can quite clearly see a big piece of steak. So I pull out my mini-hoover and suck out the gravy, before pulling out my special forceps and fishing out the offending item. We ventilate the patient and a couple of minutes later he's sat up talking. We help the guy up and put him in a wheelchair, and as we're pushing him towards the exit, the whole restaurant erupts into cheering and clapping. I feel like an actor leaving the stage after a triumphant opening night, or a golfer walking off the eighteenth green after winning the Open.

I resist the temptation to wave on my way out, but I'm not going to pretend I didn't enjoy it. It was a nice bit of impromptu theatre for the crowd. As for the patient, he returned two hours later to finish his meal. Not really. But you can bet your life one of his mates took him home a doggy bag.

14

STORING UP PROBLEMS

Not long after I started working for the ambulance service, a colleague said to me, 'Are you in a relationship?'

'Yeah.'

'I give it a few months.'

I didn't know what he was on about. I soon found out.

When I was twenty-one, I met Amy. We got on like a house on fire, made each other laugh and had a perfect friendship. The friendship grew, we ended up in a relationship and I thought, *She'll do nicely. I'll ask her to marry me.* I decided to do things properly and ask her dad's permission, and I will never forget the walk up his driveway: it was only about 10 metres long but felt more like 10 miles. Thankfully, he gave me his blessing and liked my plan, which was to ask her while we were on holiday in Egypt, on my birthday.

But I couldn't wait that long. One night, with the help of my future sister-in-law, who was also on holiday and in on the plan, I kitted out our hotel balcony with candles, led Amy out there, went down on one knee . . . and lost the power of speech. I think the penny dropped when I fished a ring from my back pocket. She said yes.

My mum and dad went out of their way to make our wedding the best day ever, as did Amy's, who are also amazing people. They helped us out with money, so that we were able to afford things we wouldn't otherwise have been able to. After what I'd been through in my previous relationship, I think they were just desperate to make me happy.

I slept terribly the night before but woke up to a belting summer's day. My old mate Neil was my best man and probably upset a few of the old folks with a joke about buying me a wedding present of some silver condoms, so I could come second for a change. But me and Amy loved it, the kids loved it and the whole day just felt perfect. I felt strong back then and knowing the family unit had been cemented made me feel even more secure.

Alas, the honeymoon in Cancún wasn't so great: it hosed it down for ten of the fourteen days and Amy got a dose of Montezuma's revenge, which confined her to bed for a week. I found myself watching daytime American TV and ordering room service, while it was chucking it down outside and Amy was writhing and groaning on the bed next to me.

We'd been married for about eight months when Amy fell pregnant. I already had three girls, so really wanted a boy. And even though I was only twenty-two, this felt like the last chance saloon. I'm sure my parents hoped so. I got my wish. And when Harrison was born, he immediately became my best mate. I was determined that whatever happened previously, any mistakes I made, wouldn't happen again. I was going to be the best dad ever for this little lad.

But when you work in the ambulance service, it's very difficult to lead a normal family life. We give an awful lot of ourselves. We work long hours and unsociable shifts, which makes us unreliable. We're often not home when we say we will be. And when we finally walk through the front door, we might be carrying a lot of mental baggage from whatever it is we've seen that day. We also miss anniversaries, birthdays of partners and kids, christenings and school plays. Compared to some hospital doctors, who work such ludicrously long hours it's scary, ambulance people have it easy. But it still makes me feel guilty. I'll explain to the kids that I can't be at this or that because there are people who need my help. And hope their nan and grandad can go instead.

You might think that I'd rush home after reeling in a drowning man from the sea or saving a choking man in a carvery, burst through the door and describe the story chapter and verse to anyone within earshot. I'm sure there are some people in the ambulance service like that. But I've never wanted to come across as if I think my job is more worthy than anyone else's.

Partners of ambulance people also go to work or stay at home with the kids, which is no picnic. They might have had a bad day, partly because their ambulance worker husband or wife has turned up late again and they've had to feed and bath the kids and put them to bed. Again. So they might want to spill their heart out about what a nightmare it's been: Johnny wouldn't eat his dinner, Sally punched Billy, Billy did a poo in the bath. That sort of thing. Everyone has their own stresses, and everyone's stresses are important to them.

Sometimes I'd listen to my wife's woes – about the new printer she'd bought that wasn't working properly, or the fact that they'd stopped stocking milk in the office fridge – and be groaning inside. But outwardly, I'd act as interested as I could: 'You're joking? No milk? Grrr. These people . . .' And once she'd offloaded, I didn't want her to think I was trying to trump her – 'Well, let me tell you what happened to *me* today . . .' It would be difficult to hold my tongue at times. But I also knew that if I lost my rag, I'd *really* lose my rag. It would be like a volcano erupting, and probably not very pretty.

Not that I'd have time to chat anyway, because I had my own responsibilities around the house. But while it's difficult knowing what to leave at work and what to bring home with you, what's certain is that not talking stores up problems. It seems easier to put your stories in a box and forget about them. But that box doesn't disappear, it sits on a shelf in a dark corner of your mind, until one day it bursts open and everything comes tumbling out in a mess.

The ambulance service defines its workers. That's why a lot of ambulance staff hook up with colleagues, because they're the only people who fully understand. Who else would know what it's like to give CPR to a baby? Or to a woman who's been flung from a moped? Or bring a drowned man back to life? That's also why I've seen so many colleagues' relationships fail, because the life of an ambulance person can seem so alien and all-consuming.

If someone told me they'd met an ambulance person and were thinking about taking the relationship to the next level, my simple advice would be: 'Make sure you know what you're getting yourself into. Make sure to give them time to unwind after work and understand that they desperately want to be at that play or birthday party.'

Sometimes the job can blindside you, which is why being able to talk to someone is really important. Just because you feel fine one minute doesn't mean you'll be feeling fine the next.

———

A job appears on our screen: ROAD TRAFFIC ACCIDENT, YOUNG MAN NOT BREATHING. We are directed to a remote country lane, where we find a cyclist on the ground, next to his bike. He isn't breathing and his heart is doing nothing at all. He has no apparent injuries and his bike is fine, so it doesn't appear that a vehicle has hit him. We can only assume that he'd been cycling along, had a cardiac arrest, toppled off his bike and died.

As with the Bolton Wanderers footballer Fabrice Muamba, who had a cardiac arrest on the pitch a few years back, this could have been down to something called cardiomyopathy, which is a disease of the heart muscle that makes it harder for a heart to pump blood to the rest of the body. Whatever it is, ambulance people can't turn up to a job with a defeatist attitude. This stricken cyclist must only be about twenty, so we're going to give it everything we have. An ambulance car soon turns up and we also radio for an air ambulance. Between us, we work on this guy for over an hour on the side of the road. There is no point in putting him in the ambulance and racing him to hospital, because administering CPR in the back of a moving ambulance is virtually impossible. Alas, ambulances don't have specially calibrated suspensions, so the journey alone can be enough to finish someone off. Imagine trying to juggle while standing up in the back of a delivery van, hurtling round corners at 70mph, and you get the idea.

We put tubes down the guy's throat, give him loads of CPR, oxygen and all the drugs we can, but it reaches the stage when we have to think about calling it off. We never like to call anything off, certainly not an attempt to resuscitate a young man. But there comes a time on any job when logic must take over from emotion. We get a senior person on the phone, tell him what we've done to try and save the patient, he considers the facts and tells us we can consider terminating resuscitation. By this time, the patient is in the back of the ambulance, and nobody wants to be the first person to step away. But eventually we have to concede that the poor lad is beyond saving.

After we've made the decision to cease CPR on the cyclist, we could quite easily discover his identity. He has a phone in his pocket, which can be unlocked using his thumbprint. So we have the discussion: should we use his thumb to unlock his phone, so that we can inform his next of kin? Or would that be breaching his confidentiality? I think it's just thinking outside the box, but one of my colleagues points out that emergency workers have been disciplined for doing it in the past, so we decide against it (I should say here that everyone should set up their medical ID on their phone, which means potentially life-saving information about allergies and medical conditions appear on your lockscreen for anyone to see without needing a password).

When you're administering CPR, you're not really looking at the patient's face. Well, you might be, but in that moment they're just a generic human being who desperately needs your help. You find your rhythm and do what you have to do. But on the way to the mortuary, it suddenly dawns on me that I know the cyclist: he's the brother of a good friend of mine.

Watching my mate's brother being placed on the mortician's table, slid into the fridge and tagged up, I'm in a daze. This is the first time I've treated someone I know. Or, more strictly, someone I used to know. And it's a terrible feeling. I don't feel like it's my place to inform his brother that I was there when he passed away. It's a grey area, there is no textbook guidance on a situation like that. Not that I had much time to weigh up my dilemma. Me and my partner left the mortuary, grabbed a brew, didn't drink it and went straight to another job.

It wasn't until about a year later that I told my mate I was on the scene when his brother passed away. I apologised for not telling him earlier and explained that I didn't know if it was best – for me and for him – if he knew. Thankfully, he understood. And he took great comfort from knowing that me and my colleagues did everything we could to try and save him. We were about five pints in at the time, which made the conversation that much easier.

I'd once told myself, 'The day I zip up a bodybag containing someone I know is the day I'm finished with this job.' But the morning after trying to save my mate's brother's life, I was back on the beat, plodding on and pretending as if nothing had happened. Carrying on and keeping calm. But only on the outside.

———

Sometimes when someone asks me what I do for a living, I'll make something up. I might say I work in a call centre or own an ice cream van. Because if I tell them I work for the ambulance service, there's a good chance the next question will be, 'What's the worst thing you've ever seen?' That's not something I really want to go into while I'm trying to have a quiet drink down the pub or at a wedding. Usually, I'll say something like, 'Believe me, you really don't want to know.' If they persist, I might fob them off with a moan about the lack of breaks we get. They tend to be less interested after that.

People have morbid curiosities. That's why there is such a huge interest in violent crime and serial killers and the like. I think there is also an assumption that because we signed up for the job, we don't have a problem seeing the terrible things we do. But what if I was honest with them? 'Well, there was the time someone plonked a child in my arms and she was covered in bruises and I could feel her broken bones clicking.' Where do you go from there?

People don't mean anything by it, it's just natural inquisitiveness. But they should remember that the person they're talking to might be horribly scarred by the worst thing they've ever seen. It's like going up to a soldier and asking how many people they've seen blown up. The last thing we want to be doing is reliving our nightmares on a night out with someone we barely know.

A colleague said to me once, 'Working as an ambulance person is like compiling a book of stamps. Most jobs will fill a little corner of a page, some jobs will fill a whole page. And when the book is full, the job's not for you any more.' Before or after an ambulance person bows out, they really don't want to be flicking through that book with Joe Bloggs down the pub. But they should be able to flick through it with a mental health professional. And when you're talking to a mental health professional, you're 'allowed' to break down and cry. That's not ideal when you're propping up the bar in Wetherspoons.

What's funny is, when I give talks in schools (which I absolutely love, but don't get paid for), they ask a lot of the same stuff as adults. Little boys, just like grown men, will ask how fast my ambulance goes (not much more than 90mph, unless you're going downhill with the wind behind you. Although I tell them it goes as fast as Lewis Hamilton's car). And they'll also want to know the worst thing I've seen. That suggests a morbid curiosity about what can go wrong with a body is inbuilt in humans. But when a little kid asks that question, I'll tell them that I once saw someone being sick. And if I really want to give them a thrill, I'll tell them that I once saw someone being sick twice.

It would make a funny scene in a film. Imagine an ambulanceman, perhaps played by Will Ferrell, at the front of a class full children, sat cross-legged on the floor. One of the kids puts their hand up and asks, 'What's the grossest thing you've ever seen?'

Ferrell smiles and replies, without skipping a beat, 'Well, only last week, I was called out to a multiple pile-up. One man had been decapitated and his friend had been thrown through the windshield . . .'

Cut to children crying, before a stern-looking teacher jogs over and cuts the ambulanceman off. Don't worry, I'd never say that to a classroom of kids. But I sometimes feel like saying it to adults who should know better.

15

THE Q WORD

There is a superstition in the ambulance service that if anyone says the word 'quiet', the shit will suddenly hit the fan. So we call it 'the Q word', just as actors refer to *Macbeth* as 'the Scottish play'. But there must have been a lot of ambulance workers forgetting themselves of late, because the shit is hitting the fan every day. I can't pinpoint exactly when it was, but someone seemed to flick a switch and things got ludicrously busy. It hasn't calmed down since.

When I first started answering the calls in the control room, it would get to 3 or 4 a.m. and there wouldn't be one job on the screen, across the whole county. Now, at 3 or 4 a.m. the screen is full of calls. The population has gone up, but not by that much. And people can't suddenly

186

be getting sicker en masse. We seem to have been hit by a perfect storm. Many of the reasons are political, and this is not meant to be an overtly political book. Suffice to say that the state of the ambulance service scares me. When that ambulance arrives, I guarantee you will get the best treatment possible. But will it arrive too late?

The last thing I want is for people to think I'm moaning about my lot. But I would at least like people to understand what us ambulance people go through. Maybe then people might think twice about swinging a punch when we walk through their front door or threatening to kill us because Mrs Miggins next door has had a stroke and we've parked an ambulance across their drive.

In an average working day, which can sometimes be part of a sixty-hour week, I might do ten different jobs. That works out at about 200 patients a month, and 2,400 patients a year. That means that over fifteen years, I've seen something like 36,000 patients. Maybe one in a hundred jobs could be classed as particularly traumatic – seeing someone die, being attacked – which comes to well over 300. Ambulance people are supposed to help, but often we're in pieces ourselves.

Last Christmas, I was lucky, because I had Christmas Day and Boxing Day off. However, I had to do a run of sixty hours between Boxing Day and New Year, during which I attended three suicides. After each one, I went home to my family, put a happy face on and pretended like nothing had happened. But while I was tucking into my leftover turkey, I couldn't help thinking about the guy I'd just seen, whose life had got so bad that he'd attached a piece of rope to a rafter in his loft, tied it around his neck and jumped through the hole in the ceiling. When I walked up the stairs, the first thing I saw were his legs, swaying from side to side. When we pulled him down, his head was facing the wrong way. Money troubles, apparently.

About a month before that, I was called to a hanging on the roof of a pub. I'm not sure what they thought we'd be able to do about it, because he'd been there since the summer. He was only found when the ceiling sprang a leak and a contractor went up to investigate an old elevator shaft, in which he made his grisly discovery. Nobody seemed to know who he was or how he got up there.

Sometimes in my job, reality merges with fiction. I look back and think, *That can't have actually happened*. But in the case of this hanged man, I'm absolutely certain of what I saw, the details of which are just too graphic to share with you. His toes were resting on the floor, so I'm almost certain there was no way of moving him without his head falling off. I didn't hang around to find out, but some poor bastard from the funeral parlour would have had to do it. It was one of the most messed-up things I've ever seen. It would certainly take a sick mind to imagine it.

As I was climbing back down the ladder, a manager shouted up, 'Lads, you shouldn't be working at heights! Health and safety!' If only he was as worried about the toll the grisly scene we'd just been exposed to might have taken on our minds.

There are some diehards who love the job so much that they won't leave until they absolutely have to, but people are leaving the ambulance service in droves. From when I started at my station, there is probably about 10 per cent of the original staff left. Some retired naturally, some left to be a paramedic or technician elsewhere. Paramedics can work in GP surgeries, police stations, call centres (although most people who went off to work for 111 came back pretty damn quick), on cruise ships and oil rigs. And most of those posts will be better paid.

Then there are those who left for a different job entirely, simply because working for the ambulance service left them at the end of their tether. Some remember the days when there would even be time for the occasional chat in the station. A moment to switch off. A moment to breathe. They started pining for those halcyon days and hating a job they once loved.

Now we're hitting the staffing targets again. But the staffing targets aren't high enough. Over the previous six years, the number of incidents classified as most serious increased by 50 per cent, while the number of paramedics increased by just 16 per cent. In Parliament in 2018, it was revealed that in my own ambulance service, one in four ambulances attending the most serious incidents do not have a paramedic on board.

Community first responders (CFRs) were never supposed to be direct replacements for ambulance workers. But when me and my colleagues first heard stories about ambulance services in other parts of the country exploring the possibility of using community first responders to drive 999 ambulances, there were conspiracy theorists who thought the time would soon come when they'd be delivering emergency treatment on the frontline, side by side with us. Thankfully, that never did happen.

CFRs are volunteers trained to provide first aid and immediate life support before a paramedic or technician can arrive on the scene. I know one CFR whose day job is testing fighter jets. As if that's not stressful enough. They provide an invaluable service in rural areas, which might be half an hour from an ambulance station, and I've actually been out to a job where a CFR has saved a life. It was a cardiac arrest on a caravan park in the middle of nowhere and by the time we got there, the patient was sitting up. My immediate thought was, *He can't have had a cardiac arrest.* But when we looked at the CFR's defib, it showed it had delivered a shock. I should probably point out that this CFR happened to be in the caravan next door, but it demonstrated just how important quick defib and CPR are.

But CFRs shouldn't exist to plug staffing gaps in ambulance services. It would be mad enough having them drive 999 ambulances – would you want a volunteer driving you to hospital in a blue-lit ambulance if you'd had a heart attack? – but the real fear is that they'll eventually become de facto initial responders, especially in rural areas. If that happens, you can bet your life that they'll be popping up in cities in no time.

In the past, ambulance crews would wait for 999 calls, and it's still the public perception that they'll dial 999 and an ambulance will come flying out of the station, like the Batmobile from the Batcave, and be on their doorstep in seconds. But we're so extraordinarily busy nowadays that 999 calls wait for the ambulance most of the time, which means you might have to wait longer than you think.

When you phone an ambulance, your needs will be graded by a system that determines urgency, called triage. Response times are divided into categories. The first category means the job is immediately life threatening – for example, a cardiac arrest – and that we should be on the scene within eight minutes. The second category means the job is serious but not immediately life threatening – a stroke, chest pains – and that we should be on the scene within nineteen minutes. The bottom category means non-life threatening – an itchy arm, a nettle sting – and that we should get there as soon as we can.

Have a quick google and you'll find desperate tales about pensioners lying for hours on pavements with broken pelvises and people waiting for hours in crashed cars. There was a story in the paper recently about a woman who fell and broke her hip. Her son travelled 200 miles from London to Devon and beat the ambulance to the scene by fifty minutes. This poor lady had been on a cold conservatory floor for seven hours, even though the ambulance station was ten minutes away. There hadn't been a mix-up, and it wasn't the fault of the frontline ambulance staff or managers, because they can only provide a service with the resources they're given. And they are unable to predict when there will be a spike in activity.

I always treat every patient how I'd want members of my family to be treated. And if a member of my family called 999, I'd expect an ambulance crew to be there in minutes. So I understand why people get annoyed when we turn up late. And whenever we do arrive late, we're immediately on the back foot. We'll pull into the patient's road and see people pacing up and down in front of their house, looking at their watch, so we immediately know they're annoyed before we even get out of the ambulance. That's not ideal.

Only the other day, a patient was kicking off because we

turned up later than we should have: 'You've broken the law! You were supposed to be here within eight minutes! It's absolutely disgusting! I'm gonna sue you! I'm gonna sue you both!' Eventually I said, 'I'm sorry you've had to wait, but we're here to help you. Please let us do that.' He kept going on and on, so I said, 'Look, we're not the complaints department. Let us do what we have to do and if you still want to complain, we'll give you the number you need.'

Presumably, this guy thought we'd seen his call on our screen and said, 'Let him wait. We'll potter over there once we've finished this brew.' He apologised in the end. Before saying he was still going to complain. But despite his lack of awareness, he had a point, and just desperately wanted to vent his frustration. When your internet goes down and you need someone to shout at, it's the poor person in the call centre who gets it in the neck, even though it's got nothing to do with them. And it's much the same when we turn up late. We take the flak without complaint, but we're doing the best we can.

What do you say to the parents of a child who has been having a fit for an hour? What do you say to an elderly gentleman, someone who fought in the war or spent his working life serving his community, who has tripped on the stairs and soiled himself while waiting for an ambulance to turn up? The whole situation is terrible for the person who needs help, and shocks the public, but it's not great for ambulance staff either.

Winter 2017–18 was particularly shocking. It's not just people falling over on the snow and ice that create those 'winter pressures' you hear about on the news, it's the so-called seasonal illnesses. Certain infections are more common when it's cold, particularly flu, which can be lethal to vulnerable people, such as the elderly, and norovirus, which is so contagious it's been known to close entire wards. Throw in chest infections and the sad fact that a lot of people, many of them old and frail, can't afford to heat their homes, and winter can send an A&E department into near meltdown.

Handovers (by which I mean handing over a patient to A&E staff at the hospital) are meant to be done within fifteen minutes, but handover times were a lot longer in the winter of 2017–18. Crews were waiting in corridors with patients on stretchers for hours. We can't just dump a patient in a corridor. We'd never want to do that anyway, but there is also a practical consideration in that we only have one stretcher, and we only get it back when the patient is found a bed. So when there are no beds available, we stand and wait.

I've heard stories of colleagues waiting for four or five hours. One shift, almost every ambulance person from my station was at the hospital. The corridors were packed with stretchers and wheelchairs, each accompanied by two ambulance crew. And while we were standing around and waiting, who was available to be sent to emergencies?

Standing around in a hospital corridor is a break of sorts, but it's not as if we can eat there. It's not uncommon not to have eaten for ten hours, or even had a cup of tea, because we're waiting to hand over patients, job after job after job. It's soul-destroying. We'd far rather be out on the road, trying to save lives. And while we wait, we're all thinking the same thing: *This is bloody appalling.* People will be rolling their eyes and making small talk, trying their best to ignore the elephant in the room. But we try to remain stoic.

It's embarrassing and stressful for all the staff involved, including us, the nurses, the doctors and even the directors, who are in a very difficult situation. Our patients are in pain and desperate to see a doctor. We've told them that they need to come to hospital, and when they turn up, they end up lying in a corridor for hours. While I'm not aware of anyone dying in a corridor on my patch, I've seen people deteriorate. And I've never seen anyone get better. Certainly, people have died while waiting in corridors in other parts of the country. In 2017, two patients died while lying in a corridor at Worcestershire Royal Hospital. One had been waiting for thirty-five hours before she died of a heart attack, which is not what she went in for.

Over the years, I've got to know a lot of A&E staff very well and they are just amazing people. Some of them have always worked in A&E, always will work in A&E and I've become good friends with them. That said, I'm making fewer and fewer friends who are doctors and nurses, because the turnover of A&E staff seems to be as high as it is in the ambulance service. But friends or not, they understand our role, we understand their role and we do everything we can to help each other out. We're all just cogs in the same giant machine.

Because I'm currently studying for a paramedic diploma, I've been spending a lot of time working in A&E, inserting cannulas in patients, taking blood and a thousand other things. And working alongside A&E staff has made it abundantly clear what immense strain these people are under. While an ambulance person normally only has one patient to deal with at a time, A&E doctors and nurses might be dealing with four or five at once. Meanwhile, there might be a queue of patients snaking out the door. A&E has always been a stressful environment, but the pressure the staff are under appears to be getting worse and worse.

When it's a Saturday night and it's standing room only in the waiting room, people are lying on stretchers in corridors and abuse and punches are flying, it's the doctors, nurses, healthcare assistants, cleaners, security guards, receptionists and people doing jobs you didn't even know existed who are keeping the plates spinning. But while it would be very easy, even understandable, for A&E staff to treat patients impersonally, as if they were sausages being fed through a machine, they still manage to treat patients with the utmost care and respect. Their dedication to the job is unwavering, despite the workload, the hours, the abuse and the pay.

———

At my interview for the job as an emergency technician, the manager behind the desk said, 'You're a young lad, if you join now, you'll be able to retire at fifty-eight.' But now the retirement age for ambulance clinicians has risen to sixty-seven, which is seven years later than police officers and firefighters. Previously, an ambulance person might have reached the age of forty-five and thought, *I've only got another thirteen years, I've got a family to keep, kids at university, I can last out until retirement.* Now that same person might think, *There's no way I can last until I'm sixty-seven; I'll have to leave and find another for ever job now, while I'm still young enough.*

———

The ambulance service is losing so many experienced paramedics and technicians, because, for many, working in the ambulance service is no longer a lifetime's vocation, it is a stepping stone to other things. And while an area losing three or four frontline staff a year might not sound like much, that might be sixty years' experience of saving lives.

I've heard of a qualified paramedic leaving to become a train driver. He was very well educated, very good at his job, but has a family to look after. He's now earning almost 60 grand a year, which is more than twice what he was earning before. I have other friends who were forced to retire in their fifties, too late to find another career, and are now scratching around trying to make ends meet. One mate retired and is now stacking shelves in Morrisons.

I'm struggling to do the job in my mid-thirties, so there's no way I'm going to last until I'm sixty-seven. The oldest partner I've had was in his early sixties. Not only did he struggle with the physical side of the job, he also struggled to keep up with technological advances and equipment and procedural changes. Maybe there are 67-year-olds who are capable of doing it, but not many. And not me. Most of the job is about communicating, and there is equipment nowadays to lessen the physical strain. But there is no getting away from the fact that the job still involves long hours and a lot of heavy lifting. An ambulance person in action can resemble a packhorse. Oxygen tanks, defibrillators and bags brimming with gear weigh a ton. I try to keep myself in decent nick, but my back is knackered, just as almost every ambulance person's back is knackered. And after we've lugged all our equipment to wherever it needs to be, we then have to treat someone, which can be exhausting in itself.

I recently went to a cardiac arrest and the patient was pretty big, and we don't discriminate against size. It's not like we can turn up and say, 'Nah, sorry love, you're too heavy. Good luck anyway.' So there were four of us carrying this lady out on a board and just as I turned to see where the step was, I missed it and fell.

It should go without saying that my female colleagues are just as capable as my male colleagues, and often fitter and stronger. But prejudice, most of it unintentional, still exists among the public. I've been on a job with a female partner and the patient has started having a go at me for 'making' her carry equipment. This old fella was flat on his back, having just had a suspected heart attack, but still had the energy to chide me for my lack of chivalry.

I've dealt with other patients who couldn't get their head around the fact that a woman was going to carry them down the stairs: 'You can't do that, you're nine stone wet through. You'll have to get your mate up here.'

Sometimes I'll reply, 'The ambulance service is an equal opportunity employer, it doesn't discriminate. Women want to be treated the same as men, and they're treated the same as men.' And a bloody good job they are, otherwise my back would be even more knackered than it is.

16

A Scary Feeling

When I started in the ambulance service, there was a snooker table in the station. We even had film Sundays, where a few of us would sit around and watch a DVD. The odd crew would go out, deal with a job and often be back in time for the end. That's how it should be. It's an extremely stressful job. We could be called to a dying child or road traffic accident at any moment. So I don't think anyone would begrudge us taking a bit of time out to process our thoughts and catch our breath.

Plus, there were other things that we could get on with at the station. Those breaks allowed us to prepare our vehicles properly. Now that the calls wait for us, we don't have time to go to the toilet, let alone make sure our ambulances are shipshape and Bristol fashion. It's not uncommon to be on a job, open a bag and discover something is missing. There are excess supplies in the back of the ambulance, but it's not ideal having to say to your patient, 'Sorry old chap, back in a minute ...' Proper prep is arguably the most important part of any job. If a soldier went into battle without squaring his kit and something went wrong, he'd be hauled over the coals.

You see those signs on the motorway: TIREDNESS CAN KILL. TAKE A BREAK. That makes perfect sense. So why would you expect an ambulance person to work for ten or more hours without pulling over for a coffee and a KitKat? The official rules state that we are entitled to a thirty-minute break during a twelve-hour shift, plus another twenty-minute one. If you're organised, you bring a packed lunch in, but often you don't get a chance to sit down and eat it. Often, I'll find myself driving the ambulance with a sweaty butty hanging out of my mouth. They say that's why our ambulances are automatics (although they're going back to manuals, and when that happens we won't even have a spare hand to eat with).

If we are able to make it back to base, by the time we've heated something up in the microwave, served it up and eaten it, we have to be straight back out the door again, probably while still chewing. You can spot ambulance people a mile off in restaurants (not when they're on shift!), because they'll be eating twice as fast as everyone else.

An ambulance person never knows when they're going to see the porcelain next, which means I do a lot of panic weeing. If I make it back to the station, I'll try to squeeze two or three wees out. If I'm in A&E, I'll try to have a couple of wees. I usually ask if I can have a wee in a patient's house. Whenever and wherever I can possibly wee, I try to sneak at least one in.

I've been on many shifts when I've been thinking, *I'm really not feeling up to the job today.* It's a scary feeling. The body is tired, the mind is tired and you're walking around with the screensaver on. Suddenly you're driving 5 tons of ambulance at tear-arse speed on the way to a cardiac arrest with a load of drugs in your bag that need to be administered properly. You arrive at a scene and start second-guessing yourself. Did I do that right? Did I forget something? When you're knackered, regulation tasks can suddenly become fiendishly difficult, whether it's doing a quick crossword or applying a dressing to a wound. At times like that, an ambulance person relies on their partner to pull them through. If you're both knackered, you just have to dig as deep as you can.

I actually have a funny story relating to fatigue. A few of my colleagues used to claim our station was haunted by a child who was trampled by an elephant. Apparently – and there is absolutely no proof that this is the case – the station is on the site of a Victorian circus. One night, a colleague claimed he couldn't get out of his chair, because there was an invisible force holding him down (I'm not sure if he thought it was the child or the elephant). Either way, his mates were quick to point out that he'd just worked ten hours without a break or anything to eat, and the invisible force was probably chronic lethargy.

No wonder we have a phenomenon in the ambulance service known as 'bell tension'. Bell tension occurs on the rare occasions you're in the station and you're watching the seconds tick down to the end of your shift. You'll be staring at the clock, pacing the room, getting a bit clammy, hoping beyond hope that another job doesn't come in and you can get home on time. Sometimes, I'll be able to hear the *Countdown* music in my head.

When it gets to about five minutes left, we'll start putting gear away – apprehensively, because we don't want to tempt fate. But that doesn't always do the trick. Once, there were literally five seconds to go when a job came in. It was a category one response (a patient was gasping for breath, and once someone in the control room hears the word 'gasping' they immediately send an ambulance) and we were the only vehicle available. It can be frustrating, but it's what we signed up for. It doesn't matter if that one last job means we end up working a fourteen-hour shift, if someone needs saving, we'll hop to it.

To add to the stress, an ambulance person's paperwork

has to be as good at 5 a.m. as at 5 p.m., even if we're so tired that we can barely see the page and the pen feels weird in our hand. Essentially, we have to show that we had a positive effect on a patient, and left them in less pain than before we arrived. I understand the need for good record-keeping, especially because people are so litigious nowadays. But it often takes as long to do the paperwork as it does to assess the patient. So you're damned if you do, damned if you don't.

It's the same for doctors. Whichever A&E department we walk into, we see them tapping away at computers, typing up their reports. That's no fault of theirs, they're just doing what they've been told to do. But, as with ambulance people, it takes up so much of their precious time and keeps them from what they're really meant to be doing, which is treating patients and saving lives.

The bosses have tried to trim our form-filling back as much as they can, but it's still quite in-depth. A cardiac arrest is one of the easier jobs to do a report for, but it gets more complicated if you leave someone at home with a chest infection. We have to explain what's wrong with the patient and what we've done to help them. We've got to speak to a doctor, and it might take ages for the doctor to call us back. Whenever he or she does, we then have to write up their findings and advice. I've been sat in a patient's living room looking at my colleague, while the patient was looking at me and we were all looking at our watches and the clock on the wall and coughing and shifting awkwardly. Sometimes, it's nice to be able to sit down and have a brew and a chat. But there are houses you don't want to spend too much time in. You just want to do what you're there to do and get out of Dodge as quick as you can.

We never know when we'll be hit with a complaint, because there's a never-ending list of things we can do wrong. On one job, we picked a guy off the floor, walked him around his living room, asked him if he was in any pain and when he said no, we said our goodbyes and left. A month or so later, the bosses received a letter of complaint from the guy's daughter, because it had been discovered that her dad had a hairline fracture of his femur.

The fact was, the patient said he was fine and was walking around, so who were we to question it? That's why before we leave someone's house, we always say, 'If you notice any changes or have any concerns, call your doctor or 999.' Me and my partner submitted written statements and, until the bosses confirmed that we'd done nothing wrong, I lived in fear of the consequences. That fear of being disciplined or dismissed is always at the back of an ambulance person's mind. It stems from the blame culture that exists in society. It's not that easy to get sacked, but the fear is very real.

Medicine is often a matter of opinion, particularly when

you don't have all the facts in front of you, which is usually the case in my job. We can have a look at a patient's blood pressure, heart rate, blood sugar levels, oxygen levels and do an ECG reading. And on the back of all that, we decide whether they should be left at home or taken to hospital. But just as we don't wear capes, neither do we have magic wands or x-ray eyes. An ambulance worker will do thousands of jobs in a year, and it's impossible to get it right every time. We're humans, so sometimes we miss things. People will argue that if an ambulance person always carries out a thorough assessment, they'll never get it wrong. Frankly, that's nonsense, because no person or system is infallible.

It doesn't matter what you do for a job, whether you're a plumber or work in a supermarket, you're going to make mistakes. The difference being, if someone stacks a shelf wrong, some boxes might fall on the floor, while mistakes made by medical professionals can have catastrophic consequences. Sometimes they're not even mistakes, they're unavoidable outcomes.

Intubating – or putting tubes down people's throats – is an art. In the ambulance service, it's a skill reserved for paramedics and the last resort for patients who are not breathing . But anaesthetists purposely put people to sleep and take over their airway management, which is a hell of a responsibility. Recently, while I was doing some training,

I offered to help an anaesthetist with a patient's airway. The patient was having her gallbladder removed and, before she arrived, me and the anaesthetist discussed the different drugs he uses as a muscle relaxant, to facilitate intubation. He explained that his favourite is rocuronium, because there is a reversal for it which can be used if the patient has an adverse reaction. Naturally, I asked him if any of his patients had had an adverse reaction, and he told me that while adverse reactions do occur, it was very rare.

This patient turned up and we had a bit of a chinwag, before the anaesthetist gave her a dose of numerous medications, including rocuronium, and off she nodded. I started to ventilate her (which basically involves squeezing an air bag connected to a mask, to inflate the patient's lungs), but it soon became a bit tricky. The anaesthetist, probably thinking my technique was awry, took over the reins, but the next thing we knew, the woman was having bronchospasms – in other words, an adverse reaction to the rocuronium, which meant she was having trouble breathing. The anaesthetist administered the reversal drug, as well as others, only for the patient to go into cardiac arrest. He pulled the emergency cord and what seemed like every medical professional in the hospital arrived within a few seconds. If you're going to have a cardiac arrest, this was the place to have it.

When the patient had been stabilised, the anaesthetist said to me, 'You're not coming in my theatre again, mate.' The patient spent a couple of days in intensive care but came out of it hunky-dory. But it made me realise that even fourteen years of training doesn't make someone bulletproof. The anaesthetist hadn't made a mistake, and neither had I, but things sometimes go wrong. In the medical world, you can never predict what will happen next with any degree of certainty.

There is also misconception among the public about what powers we have. Paramedics and technicians aren't trained to do all the things they can do in a hospital; we're only trained to carry out certain interventions. People are pushing for paramedics to be able to carry out more complicated procedures and prescribe more drugs, which means it's an interesting time to be in the job, but deciding whether a child should be left at home or not is a huge decision and not necessarily reflected in a paramedic's pay cheque.

The other weekend, I was called to a 111 referral. We turned up at this house to find a kid with a runny nose and a cough. I had to explain to the kid's mum that we're not paediatricians. Unless a kid is having an allergic reaction, cardiac arrest or something similarly serious, it's not our area of expertise. Children are also less able to communicate their symptoms. We don't carry around x-ray machines, brain scanners and all that other shiny, expensive gadgetry in our kit bags. It's not a case of being work-shy, it's a case of making sure the right people are making often monumental, life-changing decisions.

————

I'm happy to admit that one of the things that attracted a teenage me to the job was the idea of being able to tear around the place, lights flashing and sirens blaring, with no risk of being flagged down by the police. But it's not quite like that. Ambulances are very specialised machines. They're not like cars or vans, they have a lot of intricate electronics and cabling. Our mechanics know the ambulances intimately and do what they can to keep them running smoothly, but these vehicles are working their socks off twenty-four hours a day, seven days a week. Usually, an ambulance will do a twelve-hour shift and be handed straight over to another crew for another twelve-hour shift. They do thousands of miles a week with barely a break, and some of them are about ten years old.

And you know what's funny? I once picked up a brand-new ambulance from the station with a sticker on it that said: 'Please drive carefully for the first 1,000 miles while the engine breaks in.' Imagine turning up to a job and saying, 'Sorry we're late. New ambulance, have to treat it gently ...'

Some ambulances drive like they've got square wheels. They creak and groan as if they're arthritic. You will need to know the knack just to get them off the starting block some mornings. I've had ambulances break down on me at least ten times, sometimes with patients in the back. Touch wood, it's never been anything drastic, like a cardiac arrest. But I have heard about ambulances breaking down with seriously ill patients on board. In such cases, the patient has to wait for another ambulance to be sent.

Not so long ago, before they started employing specialist teams, we'd transfer neonatal babies to specialist children's hospitals. We used a special stretcher, which was basically an incubator that clipped into the back of the ambulance and was attached to the mains. It's difficult to think of a more precious cargo. We'd want to get them to their destination as quickly as possible, while trying not to accelerate or go round corners too fast or brake too heavily. And we were acutely aware that we were driving a vehicle that wasn't always the most reliable.

To compound the problems, we don't always drive the ambulances in perfect road conditions. In winter, we can end up on roads covered in black ice and deep snow. Bad weather is a particular problem for rural ambulance crews, who rely heavily on support from Mountain Rescue. Meanwhile, the public rely on hardy carers, who think nothing of wading through a couple of feet of snow to get to patients. But I have been on shifts when the snow has been almost impassable, and in those situations, you just have to do make do and mend. The skid car training has come in handy, but just the simple act of passing other vehicles becomes a nightmare, because you don't really want to be forcing people into the deeper snow on the edges or in the middle, so that they end up stuck themselves. During the day, you can try to call in a helicopter ambulance, but that's where the extra support ends. And at night, our helicopters are out of action anyway, because reduced visibility makes it too much of a risk to fly.

One shift, we were sent to a child who was fitting. It was the middle of the night, the snow was a few inches deep on the roads and every corner we went around we'd lose the back end of the ambulance. When we finally arrived at the job, the child was even more unwell than we thought, which meant we had to get to the hospital as quick as we could. But because of the weather conditions, we were looking at the best part of forty minutes. That's a very frustrating position to be in, and one for cool heads. We knew the child desperately needed a doctor's help, but if I'd put my foot down and gone too fast, I probably would have lost it. And if we'd ended up wrapped around a lamp post or stuck in the snow, we might have never arrived at the hospital and instead been sat there for an hour waiting for another crew to relieve us. So we just had to navigate our way through the blizzard and keep everything crossed. Actually, that's not a bad metaphor for what it takes to be an ambulance person when things are getting chaotic.

17

MESSED UP AND DARK

It has been another common or garden morning when a job comes on our screen: CHILD FALLEN OVER IN SHOWER. UNCONSCIOUS. I always feel anxious whenever a child is involved. As a father of four young children, it would perhaps be strange if I didn't. At the same time, experience has taught me not to always believe what I read on the screen. So I do wonder if this child is really unconscious. Although maybe it's because I don't want it to be true.

Me and my old mate Paul are only a few miles from the house and we arrive within minutes, siren blaring and blue light flashing. The house is in a relatively deprived area on a terraced street, with cars parked all along it, which means we have to park blocking the road. No doubt we give one of the neighbours the hump. Oh well.

Usually in jobs where kids are involved, the parents are waiting on the doorstep in a state of panic, so that we have to calm them down as well as deal with the emergency at hand. Not in this case. I knock on the door. No answer. I knock again. No answer. I think to myself, *That's odd, if my kid had fallen over and knocked themselves unconscious, I'd have that door wide open so that the ambulance people could turn up and sweep straight in.*

There is a little alleyway running next to the house, so we make our way down there with all our gear on, kicking and shouldering aside weeds and overhanging branches. We reach a dilapidated wooden gate, force it open, pick our way through more weeds and piles of rubbish, bang on the back door and shout 'Ambulance!' Again, no answer.

I try the door and it's locked. By now, we're wondering if we have the right address. But suddenly, we hear the thud, thud, thud of big feet thundering down stairs. The door swings open to reveal a burly lad standing there with a limp child in his arms. Behind him, another toddler is peeping around a door. For a few seconds, the guy stands there staring at us, as if we're a couple of salesmen flogging brushes. Eventually he says, 'There you go, mate', and shoves the child into my chest, as if she is nothing more precious than a pile of dirty washing or a tray of beers.

When I look down, I can tell immediately that the girl, who is about two years old, has horrendous injuries. Her face is black and blue, as are her legs. Her eyes are half-closed, her pupils dilated and her breathing is noisy and slow, which is always a bad sign. She is also completely dry, which suggests that the story about her falling in the shower is concocted. Paul says, 'She's really poorly.' I give him a look that says, 'Let's move quick.'

We tell the guy to be as quick as he can and bring the other child with him. I hand the patient to Paul, who can feel her body clicking, which suggests she also has broken bones. We both know something is seriously amiss, but we can't say that. We just have to try to save her life and leave it to the police to establish what has gone on. Meanwhile, a couple of cars are beeping their horns, their drivers only worried about themselves, not the little girl we are trying to save. The selfishness of some people is remarkable to behold. They couldn't see exactly what we were doing, but that's besides the point.

I get on the radio and say, 'Critically ill child, unconscious. We need the full team ready to receive us.' Me and Paul have worked with each other so often that we have an almost telepathic understanding. We throw everything at her, but she soon stops breathing. I drive the ambulance to the hospital as if I've stolen it, but the journey seems to take for ever. And the whole way there I'm thinking, *This girl reminds me so much of my kids – blonde hair, blue eyes, a beautiful little thing.*

When we arrive at the hospital, there is a full crash team ready to go: nurses, doctors, consultant, anaesthetist. We tell them everything we know – which isn't very much – and what procedures we've carried out, and they take over from there. It's always a privilege to watch a group of highly trained clinicians working together, as if they're different parts of one perfectly calibrated machine. They manage to stabilise and intubate the little girl, but her injuries are such that it looks like she might go downhill very quickly. So a helicopter is called in to fly her to a specialist unit in another city. Me and Paul accompany the patient to the chopper and watch it take off, before trudging slowly back to A&E, neither of us saying a word.

Back at the hospital, the man has now been joined by the little girl's mother. The doctors have already told them that the situation is grave, but the bloke doesn't seem to be registering. The mother, on the other hand, is in a right old state. From what I can work out, the man is the mother's new boyfriend and had been looking after her kids while she was at work. The doctors agree with us that the girl's injuries are non-accidental, so I get on to the police, tell them about our suspicions and they immediately instigate a serious investigation. We provide them with statements, make our exits and a short while later, the man is arrested.

We drive to the ambulance station in stony silence. When we arrive, we both agree that we can't possibly deal with anything else that day. We've done enough, it's time to go home. In my ten years of service, I have never felt so low and utterly exhausted.

At home, I can't shake the image of the little girl in my arms, covered in bruises, wheezing and gasping for breath. She was just an innocent toddler, who should have been playing in the garden or having fun with her friends. I also can't stop thinking about the man's seediness and apparent indifference. I sit there on the sofa for hours, thinking: *What a messed-up world we live in.*

I told my wife what had happened and she took me out for tea and tried to take my mind off it. But I struggled to sleep that night. I kept playing things over and over in my mind. Had I done something wrong? Could I have done more? I could still smell the house, all burnt toast and overcooked vegetables. I could see the face of the other little girl, peeping round the door. I was assailed with images of that black and blue little body. Round and round it went.

The next day, I asked Paul how he was feeling. He seemed to be dealing with it okay. I didn't want to burden him, so I said I was fine as well. But I wasn't fine at all, I had gone into a tailspin. I sat there, staring at the telly.

Not watching, just staring. But in my head, the visions were becoming more vivid and more frenzied. When I did manage to doze off, my mind tried to put the pieces together. I could see the man hitting the screaming child, and the scene became ever more violent. I'd wake up soaked in sweat, my heart pounding. It reached the point where I was desperately fighting to stay awake instead.

After two scheduled days off, I went back to work. I was quieter than normal, tried not to make eye contact and avoided engaging. That was probably me giving uncon-scious hints that I needed help. But nobody said anything. And why would they? They probably just thought I needed a bit of time to reacclimatise after a particularly rough job.

In reality, I was rapidly descending to the bottom of a deep, dark hole and the world was passing by above my head. Unless I made a concerted effort to concentrate on whatever job was at hand, all I could see was the face of that poor battered girl. I was consumed by guilt and numb to anything that was going on around me. And when I got home, it got worse. Even the sound of the kids' feet reminded me of the man stomping down the stairs.

I'd had no training in how to deal with a situation like this and there was no one I felt I could talk to. So I hid my trauma from everyone and suffered in silence instead. I should have talked to my wife, but I didn't want to burden her with my problems. I was the man of the house and needed to get a grip and pull myself together. My wife was always happy to listen, but she didn't work for the ambulance service, so I didn't think she'd understand. When I heard that the man had been charged with grievous bodily harm, I thought that might make me feel better. But it made things worse. I grew angrier and more frustrated. Whenever I imagined his vile face, I wanted to scream.

Culturally, things hadn't changed much since the time I was stabbed as a teenager. A stiff upper lip was still seen as a noble and dignified thing to possess. If you're a bloke reading this, when was the last time a male mate said to you, out of the blue, 'How's life? Are you okay? Do you need to talk about anything?' When was the last time a male mate gave you a cuddle? Whatever the answer, it doesn't happen nearly enough. Often people don't talk because they're worried that their mates just won't get it. I suspect that's particularly the case in the services, whether you're an ambulance person, a copper or a firefighter. But doctors, nurses and soldiers will have the same dilemma.

It can be terribly deflating reaching out to someone and revealing your inner turmoil, only to be met with indifference: 'Oh, that sounds awful ... anyway, let's keep it light, shall we?' I can't really blame anyone. I'm not really interested in the nitty-gritty of other people's jobs, and I often assume they're not really interested in talking about whatever it is they do for a living either.

Sometimes, someone will ask me how work has been and I'll really want to say, 'Well . . . I'm dealing with more dead people than you can shake a shitty stick at. I went to this one bloke who was found dead on the roof of a pub. And I saw this other bloke being dragged out of his house with smoke billowing off him. I could feel the heat radiating from his body and smell his burning flesh.' Stories like that, which I experienced in every dimension and rattled me to my boots, are not easy to bring up down the Dog and Duck: 'A pint of Fosters and some Scampi Fries please, Trevor. When you get back, I'll tell you about the man I saw face down in a puddle. Then we'll have a go on the quiz machine . . .'

I became more withdrawn at work, to the extent that I almost stopped talking. I stopped playing with the kids. It was as if someone had switched me off and I was sleepwalking, which isn't ideal when you're tasked with saving people's lives. Then I heard that the girl had died and the man had been charged with murder. This pushed me further towards breaking point.

I started drinking heavily, usually on my own, to combat my anxiety and help me sleep. It didn't work. There was a three-month wait for the case to come to court, and the closer it got to the date, the more anxious I became about giving evidence. I felt such a heavy responsibility. Because I was desperate to do my best for the murdered girl, I was playing the scene over and over in my head, to make sure I didn't leave out any important details and allow this scumbag to wriggle off the hook.

I had a friend and colleague called Rich who was about my age, so I decided to reach out to him. But it wasn't easy. My original plan was to phone him, but I couldn't summon the courage. So I wrote him a text message, which I quickly deleted. I rewrote and eventually sent it, but immediately turned off my phone, because I was terrified by what he would say. When I turned it back on about half an hour later, I had a message from him: 'I'm on my way round. Put the kettle on.'

When Rich turned up I kind of broke down. I already knew what I had to do – make an appointment with my GP, speak to a counsellor – but Rich reaffirmed it. In addition, he let me know that it was okay to feel like I did, that anyone who had seen what I did might feel the same. In short, he made it very clear that he understood. That conversation was the start of the next chapter.

Two or three weeks after attending the dead child, I paid a visit to my GP, at my wife's suggestion. She offered to come with me, but I didn't want her to see me cry. Sitting in the surgery's waiting room, I was thinking, *I can't be doing with this.* And even as I was walking into the doctor's room, I was considering changing my story: 'Oh, it's probably nothing serious, but I'm a bit worried about this mole . . .' I was embarrassed. I was a man, and real men don't have these problems. And if they do, they certainly don't share them. Not only that, I was supposed to be a hardy professional, not weak and feeble.

I plonked myself down on the chair and wanted the ground underneath to swallow me up. The doctor said, 'How can I help you?' I sat in silence for maybe a minute. Eventually I said, 'I don't really know where to start. It's a long story. I work for the ambulance service, I saw something terrible. And I've been having a hard time since.' As soon as I said that, it was like the weight of the world had been lifted from my shoulders. That first step is always the hardest.

My doctor was so understanding and supportive. She signed me off work and referred me for counselling. My counsellor was an amazing guy called Roger, who was based in the same surgery, a couple of doors from my house. Roger was a former police counsellor and totally got what I was going through. But while chatting to him helped, I felt like I couldn't get well until the court case had been and gone.

However, on the day he was due to stand trial, the man changed his plea from not guilty of murder to guilty of manslaughter, which meant my evidence was no longer needed. The Crown Prosecution Service accepted his story that he'd lost his temper and violently shaken her, and he was sentenced to nine years in prison. It felt like being kicked in the stomach. I'd built myself up, braced myself, and now it felt like this guy had got away with murder.

The post-mortem examination had found that the girl had suffered severe head injuries, a lacerated liver, bruising to the lining of her stomach and other parts of her body. Her mother had been in police custody while she was dying, because her boyfriend hadn't told the truth. And the person who had caused all this suffering would probably be out in a few years.

I lost all faith in the justice system, but I had no choice but to accept the decision and try to get on with my life. But I still wasn't right. I became less and less interested in the people around me. I wrapped myself in a blanket of sorrow and all I could think about was how messed up and dark the world was.

I got the odd call from work, but the 'How are you feeling?' was usually closely followed by 'When do you think you'll be back in?' or 'Can you send another sick note?' Nobody ever said, 'Is there anything we can do to help you?' I'm sure people cared, but it didn't come across that way. If your bosses aren't telling you not to worry about not coming in, you're likely to think you're letting the side down. Like a soldier injured in battle and dragged from the field, I felt guilty that my mates were still out there on the frontline.

Mental illness doesn't just affect the person afflicted by it, it also affects the people closest to them. My wife tried to reach out to me, but I wasn't interested. And before long, my marriage was falling apart. I was there in person but not in spirit. Amy could see I was suffering and tried to help. But I shut her out, which was obviously difficult for her to deal with.

But Roger was like a port in a storm. He left no stone unturned, delved right back to even before I was stabbed. And once he'd prised open the lid, everything came pouring out. He made me realise that a life is like a house. Your foundations are the childhood your parents give you (thank God my foundations were sturdy) and each year after that is like a row of bricks. Some of those rows will be laid with crumbling bricks and iffy cement, and if you ignore those flaws and carry on building on top of them, eventually the whole house will come crashing down. That's what happened to me. Early fatherhood, the stabbing, the murdered woman, the dead child, the hangings, the drownings, the overdoses, the car crashes, the cardiac arrests, they'd all been compacted, but now they had come loose. And now it was a case of gathering up the debris and trying to make it whole again.

Roger encouraged me to channel the energy I'd not been able to use to give evidence in the court case into trying to instigate a change elsewhere. He suggested that before

I return to work, I speak to my manager. So after about four months off, when I was starting to feel a bit more like my old self, I arranged a meeting. My manager insisted that HR be there, which made me think that they were worried I was going to lodge a complaint. That was never my intention.

At the meeting, I explained that I'd attended this horrible job, which had led to me being diagnosed with post traumatic stress disorder (PTSD), and that I didn't think I'd been given sufficient support by the ambulance service. Actually, I hadn't been given *any* support by the ambulance service. My manager sympathised with me, before saying, 'If you can't cope, then maybe this isn't the job for you.'

I was quite taken aback by his response and couldn't understand why they were so reluctant to help. I thought I was worth more. I told the manager I disagreed that it wasn't the job for me and that it was more a case of me having a rough time and him needing to support me. But it was at that exact moment that I decided that if the culture within the service meant that my bosses couldn't do anything about it, then I would.

18

ROAD TO RECOVERY

Before I was diagnosed with PTSD, I thought I was infallible, hard as nails, tough as old boots. Looking back, I was quite naive. I thought that once I'd dealt with my first dead body, it would become gradually easier to deal with things.

People sometimes ask me if there had been signs that the job was affecting me and I'd ignored them. I honestly can't recall any, even in hindsight. That said, hardly anyone in the service knew what signs to look for. I'd have the odd colleague who would say to me, 'After a long day at work, I need a couple of beers or a few glasses of wine to help me switch off.' But I didn't put two and two together and it would be dishonest of me to say that I saw colleagues disintegrate before my eyes. Instead, they were there one day, gone the next.

One of the first ladies I worked with, who was a top trainer and the loveliest person you could meet, clocked off one day and I never saw her again. I heard on the grapevine that she'd hit the bottle and I didn't think to ask why. Just as in my case, the pressure had presumably built up gradually so that no one noticed, so that she was like the proverbial frog in boiling water.

It's only now that I can guess that some colleagues didn't leave the ambulance service simply because a better offer came up, but because the pressures of the job were making them ill. It wasn't really until I was diagnosed with PTSD that I realised I was vulnerable – and that everyone was vulnerable. And having made that discovery, I wanted people to know that no one is immune to mental health problems and that it is okay to have one. So the day after that meeting with management, I wrote and posted the first of many blogs, detailing my crash and subsequent road to recovery:

In the ambulance service, we like to have this feeling that we're bulletproof, and sometimes you can feel a bit ashamed to admit that there's something wrong with you. But we're humans, not robots, and I want people to know that they shouldn't be afraid to talk and seek help if they need it . . .

The main theme of the blogs was the benefit of talking, whether to your partner, your mates, your GP or a counsellor. I explained that there was no shame in events getting on top of you, and that reaching out for help was the best – albeit one of the most difficult – things I'd ever done.

Publicly admitting I had a mental health problem scared me. I honestly thought I might lose my job. And what would my colleagues think of me? Would people not want to work with me because they thought I was weak, incompetent and therefore a liability on the frontline? Would they think I might break down on the job? I didn't know how I'd cope either. I worried that I was more vulnerable than before.

As it was, though, I slipped straight back into the old routine and felt mentally stronger than I had before. They call that post-traumatic resilience or growth – or, proverbially speaking, whatever doesn't kill you makes you stronger. Some people didn't know what to say, because a colleague being off for so long with mental illness was new to them. But almost all of them treated me as if nothing had happened, so that I immediately felt like part of the gang again.

Back on the road, I worked mainly with my old buddy Paul. Those early shifts consisted mainly of bread-and-butter jobs – grannies falling over, heart attacks, fits and cardiac arrests. It was the same old hard slog with the same old stresses, but nothing overly taxing. However, I worried that if I had to deal with another child who had been seriously harmed – or worse – my world might implode again.

I'd been back on the job for a few weeks when my blogs went viral, which was a bit embarrassing. But they had the desired effect. Those blogs, and the responses to them, changed my life for ever. The proverb 'A problem shared is a problem halved' is slightly optimistic, but there is a lot to be said for it. Ambulance workers from all over the country sent me emails, thanking me for sharing my story. These were people who had been through similar things, some of whom had recovered, some of whom had been suffering in silence before reaching out to me. It's such a simple thing, having a chat with someone. But people find it so difficult. So it was great to see people taking the leap.

One of the most hardened paramedics I knew collared me and said, 'I read your blog. It was inspirational. I had a similar problem but never told anybody about it.' With that, he shared his story for the first time. It turned out he wasn't as hardened as I thought he was. Because I'd revealed my own vulnerability, others felt empowered to reveal theirs. They suddenly realised that they weren't the only ones, so were no longer embarrassed.

Becoming the go-to man for people wanting to unburden themselves was nice, but also a big responsibility. And while I could listen, I wasn't able to provide any practical help or solutions. It also confirmed that we had a long, long way to go. Why had these people been suffering in silence for so long? Was the ambulance service doing something wrong in terms of mental health support? Yes, because there wasn't any. But nobody had ever suggested that they needed to do more. There was a deep-seated culture in the ambulance service, as impenetrable as granite. Sharing my story and encouraging others to share theirs was just the start; next it was a case of getting the powers that be to take mental health more seriously.

It struck me that there was far more discussion in the media about mental illness in the military. I'm sure the military's mental health support isn't perfect, but the myriad documentaries and stories in papers and on the news about soldiers returning from Iraq or Afghanistan with PTSD had made the Ministry of Defence take notice. But the media's focus on the military gave me hope, because it demonstrated that raising awareness about an issue could lead to a change in culture. Soldiers publicly discussing mental illness sends out a powerful message, because it shows that however tough you are, you are susceptible. Our soldiers should receive as much support as possible. They're incredibly brave and selfless people who do a vital job for our country, and they must see some terrible things in war. But ambulance workers see terrible things, too. Certainly, ambulance workers deserve the same level of support.

———

A couple of months after returning to work, I'm in the ambulance with Paul and a job appears on our screen: FEMALE BLEEDING PV. PV is the abbreviation for *'per vaginam'*, or from the vagina. It's not uncommon and there is nothing in this job description to suggest it will be anything out of the ordinary. The usual process is to assess whether the patient is hypovolaemic, which is a state of decreased blood volume, specifically a decrease in plasma. Meanwhile, we do what we can to stem the bleeding and get her into hospital to see a gynaecologist as quickly as possible. But when we turn up at the address, the situation is a bit more complicated than normal.

A guy meets us at the front door and says, calm as you like, 'In here, lads.' We stop off for a quick chat with a toddler in a highchair in the living room before making our way through the kitchen and into a bathroom at the rear of the house. Sprawled in the bath is a woman. There is blood everywhere. All over the bath, all over the tiles, all over the woman. She looks like she has been drained of blood, so that her papery skin is almost transparent. She's just about able to open her eyes and talk to us, but not able to make much sense.

Despite the grisly scene, there is nothing to suggest foul play. My initial thought is that it could be a ruptured ectopic pregnancy, which is when a fertilised egg implants itself outside of the womb. Or maybe it's a miscarriage. But when I ask the guy if there was a risk of pregnancy, he replies that there wasn't. It doesn't enter my head that he could be lying to me. And whatever it is, it's not our job to find out. Instead, we slip seamlessly into battle mode.

We aren't able to get a canular into her to give her some fluids, because her body has almost completely shut down. She's unable to stand on her own, so simply removing her from the bath is a major operation. I have to move all sorts of stuff out of the way to get to her – baskets and cabinets full of toiletries, towels and toilet rolls – and sling it all in the hallway. Paul arrives with the wheelchair and I try to get a grip on her top end, which is easier said than done, because of the blood and the clamminess of her skin. Paul grabs her legs, we lift her out and how we manage to get her in the wheelchair without either of us slipping over and breaking something is a minor miracle.

We wheel her out to the ambulance, lay her on the stretcher, get the oxygen on and eventually manage to get a canular into her. But I still think there's a very good chance she'll die on the way to the hospital, because the address is probably as far from the hospital as it's possible to be. We don't even have time to wash ourselves down, so while Paul remains in the back of the ambulance with the patient, I drive to the hospital covered in blood.

Typically, it's one of those days when my fellow road-users decide to be a royal pain in the arse. Cars keep pulling out in front of me and choosing not to stop. And all the time I can feel the pressure rising. On arrival at the hospital, I slam the handbrake on, snap on some fresh gloves and open the back door. The woman looks even worse than when we first turned up at the house. But she's still alive and still saveable, which is the most important thing. We race her into the resuscitation room and hand over to the nurses and consultant. And with that, me and Paul think our part of the job is done. But while we're washing ourselves in the sink, making idle chat and thinking about doing the paperwork, cleaning up the ambulance and getting ourselves home, the consultant walks over and says, 'Paul, Dan – where's the baby?'

During his examination, the consultant has discovered a severed umbilical cord and delivered a nearly full-term placenta. But we tell him we don't know about any baby. We asked the man in the house, and he said there wasn't one. But I get this feeling in my gut that we should have probed a bit more.

I radio the police and my control room and tell them

they need to get over to the address as soon as possible, because there's potentially a baby in there somewhere. Later, I learn that the police did indeed find a baby, in a plastic bag in the hallway. Sadly, it was already dead.

If we had known there was a baby in the house, we'd have got another ambulance round there straightaway. But all we could do in the circumstances was ask the question. As it was, I wrote a statement for the police, went back to work and did a pretty good job of forgetting about it. The case didn't go to criminal court and I didn't ask why. Given what had happened before, I think colleagues were concerned what effect the job might have on me. But I didn't feel anything beyond the concern which was to be expected. Maybe it would have been different had I seen the dead baby, but it was probably more likely that I was that much more resilient.

19

WHY?

Around the same time as I was writing my blogs, the charity Mind was setting up something called the Blue Light Programme, which was also focused on raising awareness of mental health issues and improving support in the emergency services. I got involved with those guys, and there seemed to be a growing realisation that things needed to change. Meanwhile, me and my colleague Rich, who admitted to being gobsmacked when I told him about my PTSD diagnosis, launched our own campaign, Our Blue Light, which was all about encouraging people to talk about mental health and reduce the stigma.

Me and Rich organised several events to raise awareness for Our Blue Light and Mind's Blue Light Programme. They included a five-month mental health relay, during which a torch was carried by emergency service volunteers across the region, a dance competition, taking part in an LGBT pride parade and a six-day, 150-mile walk, during which we visited police, fire, ambulance and RNLI stations across the country and discussed the importance of opening up about mental health.

Four of us did the walk from start to finish, and it was the toughest thing I'd ever done, walking 25–30 miles a day, before waking up the next morning and doing it all again. But we got an amazing reception at the stations. People seemed genuinely chuffed that we were doing something to raise awareness, and some of them shared their stories of mental turmoil with us. On the final day, about 100 people walked the last 20 miles with us, which attracted journalists, who relayed our message to the public through TV, radio and newspapers.

About a year after I'd attended the lady bleeding in the bath, I received a letter from family court. The authorities wanted to take the toddler we'd seen in the house away from its mum and for me and Paul to give evidence.

I'd never given evidence in family court before and didn't know what to expect. I turned up in my uniform and wiled away the hours in the waiting room making small talk with Paul and a police officer involved in the case. But while I looked calm, I was churning up inside.

An usher came in, said it was my turn and asked if I

was okay. I told her I was fine. She led me into the court-room and said, 'See that chair over there in that box? Go and sit yourself down.' So I wandered over and plonked myself down behind this big pile of files. Suddenly, some-one shouted from the back of the courtroom in this big, booming voice, 'Stand until the judge tells you to sit!' That certainly told me. And it got worse from there.

I am not at liberty to say exactly what went on in the courtroom that day, except that nobody seemed to care that I was a nice young man who saved people's lives for a living and most of my answers were 'I'm sorry, but I don't recall'. I felt really guilty for not being able to remember, because it felt like I wasn't helping anyone, prosecution or defence. But I'd had no guidance, no one had told me what I might be asked. What else could I do but tell them the truth, which was that – over a year later – the job was little more than a smudge on the memory?

On my way out of the courtroom, me and Paul passed like ships in the night. About ten minutes later, Paul was back in the waiting room, looking as cool as a cucumber. Meanwhile, I looked like I'd just been given a going over by the Spanish Inquisition.

Paul said, 'All right, pal? That wasn't much of a prob-lem. Was it?'

I've no idea why I was given a sustained grilling and they went easy on Paul, other than to say that it was typical: Paul had a habit of making life look easy, however different the reality.

Afterwards, the copper told us that the guy who was in the house had taken his own life. I can only guess that he cut the umbilical cord, placed the baby in the plastic bag and admitted it before killing himself, which is why the case was never processed through criminal court. Why he decided to do what he did I'll never know. Meanwhile, the toddler had been placed in social care. The court hearing was to decide whether the woman would lose her child for ever. I never found out what happened, and I decided it was probably best to reserve my opinion. The mind naturally craves answers, but I was quite happy not to have them, especially while I was still going through my recovery process. Maybe that was something I'd learned to do, on an unconscious level. It wasn't my job to play judge and jury.

That job was strange but also quite typical. One minute we're on our way to a run-of-the-mill PV bleed, the next we find a woman covered in blood in a bath, the next we find out there was a dead baby on the scene, the next I was in court giving evidence about something I didn't even see.

What I haven't mentioned is how overwhelming it was to see that woman alive and well. I played a part in saving her life, and that's all that mattered. I took great comfort from the fact I'd done my job well. I could only hope that the right decisions were made for her surviving child and he or she goes on to live a happy and healthy life.

As with the case that had triggered my PTSD, I didn't really discuss the job or the subsequent court case with Paul. He was a guy who seemed happy just plodding along and I took that to mean he was a stronger person than me. We'd actually stopped working with each other nearly as much as we had done. We remained great mates but had both decided that we'd become too comfortable in each other's company and that there was a danger of us becoming complacent on the job. We also thought that spending so much time together in work might adversely affect our friendship out of it.

Not long after the court case, I found myself running around a nightclub, helping set up a reception to raise even more awareness. I was still working full-time for the ambulance service, and I'm not sure how I found the hours to organise it. But I desperately wanted it to be a great night for everyone. It was while I was scurrying around, tying up various loose ends, that I received a phone call from my manager. Paul, that immovable rock who had been by my side during some of my toughest moments, had taken his own life.

At first, I thought it was one of Paul's sick wind-ups. I wouldn't have put it past him, given some of the stories he'd told me. Then I thought my manager must have got it wrong and that another Paul had ended it all. When it finally sunk in that it was true, I was stunned. I also felt incredibly guilty and hypocritical. Paul knew what I was going through, because I decided to talk about it. But nobody knew what Paul was experiencing. When I asked him how he was coping, he said he was fine. When I told him I'd started a campaign to raise awareness of mental illness, he wished me well and said he didn't want to get involved. I didn't argue and I didn't probe any deeper. I told myself that he'd processed what he had seen and was simply a tougher man than me. But the whole time I'd been pouring my heart and soul into raising awareness of mental illness in the ambulance service, encouraging people to talk, my old mate had been sinking into an abyss which would eventually engulf him.

Why wasn't I a better friend to him? Was there more I could have done or more I could have said? I knew he had domestic problems and had been through some turbulent times, but he always appeared so unflustered and I just assumed he'd settle down eventually. I certainly didn't notice any warning signs. Maybe I wasn't looking hard enough. It's so easy to get stuck in your own little bubble and forget to look out for those around you. That's what I told myself, but it didn't make me feel any better.

I couldn't stop thinking about the last time I'd seen him, in the corridor at the station. He said to me, 'Mate, we need to get breakfast club back up and running.' And I replied, 'Definitely, I'll drop you a text next week.' I never did. How often does that happen? So often, something else is going on that seems to be more important. I wondered what he would have told me over that fry-up. Maybe if I'd given him the chance to offload his problems, he wouldn't have gone through with it. I had a million and one questions to ask, but now Paul wasn't around to answer them.

Paul's death hammered it home that the necessary help wasn't there. As I understand it, his mental illness wasn't entirely down to what he saw on that job and he had a great family around him. But if a medical professional had reached out to him and asked if he was okay, they might have got him to talk. Instead, he felt so isolated that taking his own life seemed like his only option.

I spent a few moments scrolling through the many pictures of me and Paul on my phone. Paul smoking where he shouldn't have been smoking. Paul posing in front of his ambulance, marooned on someone's front lawn. And then I had no choice but to put my grief to one side, put on a smile and get on with organising the ball.

When I spoke that night, I wasn't just speaking about me and my experiences of mental illness, I was speaking about Paul and all the other emergency service workers who had been let down by a complacent culture.

20

SOMETHING POSITIVE

After I wrote a piece about my experiences of mental illness for Mind's website, they invited me to speak at the launch of a new initiative called Heads Together on World Mental Health Day 2016. Heads Together is spearheaded by Prince Harry and the Duke and Duchess of Cambridge (or William and Kate), and the event involved lots of people sharing their stories on stage.

They were keen for me to explore the idea that one conversation can change everything. And it was that first conversation with Rich, when he dropped everything to answer his mate's SOS call, that they wanted me to talk about. The message they wanted me to convey was that however isolated you feel, and however short of friends you might be, there is always someone who can help, whether it be a colleague, a doctor or a Samaritan on the end of the phone. If only Paul had known that there were people out there who wanted to listen. People he'd never even met.

I actually had a whole network I could plug into, including my old mate Neil, my wife, my parents and even my children. So I felt slightly uncomfortable about playing down their support. But each person in a support network can't be looking out for you 24/7. They go to work, look after children, go on holiday and have their own problems to deal with. And in this case, it was Rich who best understood how great a toll an ambulance person's work can take on them and how difficult it is for them to admit vulnerability. Rich made me realise that asking for help is okay.

Heads Together had also invited people like the former England cricketer Andrew Flintoff and musician Professor Green, so I guess I was there as the 'normal' person. It was a surreal experience for an everyday working-class lad, but it was great that they wanted to use my story to get people talking and I felt good that I'd managed to turn such a scary period in my life into something positive.

While the Duchess of Cambridge was giving her spiel, it was just me and Prince Harry on the side of the stage. He knew I was on next and could tell I was nervous, so tried his best to put me at ease. It was just small talk really.

A bit of stuff about the weather and about how nervous Kate looked. But he also told me how great my story was and how important it was that I told it to as many people as possible.

I did my talk and when Harry did his, he said lots of nice things about me and that he hoped more people would talk about their problems as a result of me opening up. When he left the stage, he shook my hand, told me how important it was that I keep telling my story and asked if I fancied running the London Marathon for Heads Together. Crafty sod, he'd buttered me up and hit me at my most vulnerable. You can't say no, can you?

Harry disappeared, probably while laughing his head off that he'd pulled off the old royal mind trick, and the next thing I knew someone was taking pictures of me with a London Marathon magazine in my hands. There was no going back from there. The only problem being I was in no fit state to run anywhere. I was still partial to the odd cigarette, the only place I ran was to the bar and the marathon was in five months' time. But I left the event with a spring in my step and a sense of purpose. Just a few well-chosen words from Prince Harry had acted as fuel to get myself fit and fanned my campaigning zeal, just as a few well-chosen words from Rich had helped me back to my feet.

When I ran past Prince Harry at a Heads Together day in Newcastle, he collared me and asked me how the training was going. I couldn't believe he remembered who I was. And I made sure to thank him for inspiring me to pound the road, shift the beer belly and put a bit of lead into my pencil. We met up again on the morning of the marathon and arranged to meet again after I was done. Sadly, he went home before I finished, later than planned.

There were times that day when I thought I'd have to quit. The first five miles were fine. London was a riot of colour and noise – cheering, steel bands, people calling my name (it was written on my bib, to be fair) – and it felt like I was riding the crest of a gigantic wave. After 10 miles, I felt a bit leggy. After 12 miles, I was coming apart at the seams. All I could think was, 'There's no way I can do another 14 miles of this.' After 18 miles, I had to stop because I was completely and utterly broken. But after twenty minutes of walking/hobbling, the support of the crowd got me jogging again. Though I didn't exactly ride on their shoulders, it was more like they were dragging me along by my armpits.

At mile 20, I spotted my wife and burst into tears. She said to me, 'You've nearly done it!' I replied, 'I haven't nearly done it, I've got another six miles to go . . .' I was running on fumes, but off I popped again, walking, limping, occasionally even running. And when I saw the 25-mile marker, a wave of energy came over me and I started running my socks off. In my head, I imagine I resembled Usain Bolt over those last couple of hundred metres. In reality, I probably resembled a man pulling a fridge. But who cares really?

I completed it in about five hours, but my time was irrelevant. I ran the same number of miles as the winner. And the faster you go, the less time you're out there suffering. That's what I told myself anyway. Finishing that marathon was one of my biggest achievements. And while it might be trite to compare the suffering endured in a marathon to everyday mental strife, I was struck by the surface similarities: had people not reached out to help me along the route, there is absolutely no way I would have made it to the finish line.

In 2017, I was invited to a Queen's garden party at Buckingham Palace. But the night before it was due to take place, a bomb exploded as people were leaving a concert at the Manchester Arena. There was some talk of cancelling the garden party, but the organisers decided to go ahead with it. I think that was the correct decision. It's become a cliché, but the cancellation of events would have meant the terrorists had won. We marked the attack with a two-minute silence and the atmosphere was suitably sombre. But I felt very uncomfortable making pleasant small talk and nibbling on cucumber sandwiches while my colleagues in the emergency services and NHS were dealing with the aftermath.

Ambulance crews raced to the arena, some of them on their days off, and when they arrived on the scene they were expecting minor injuries. What actually awaited them was a vision of hell. I felt guilty that I wasn't able to help, just as a soldier feels guilty when his mates get caught up in a firefight and he's elsewhere. I just couldn't help thinking, *Why them and not me?*

There was some criticism directed at the emergency services in the aftermath of the bombing. It was claimed that the response was too slow and confused. This isn't the place to discuss such things. But what I can say, having heard some of my colleagues' stories, is that it's impossible to imagine the terrible things they saw that night and I'm incredibly proud to have all who were involved as colleagues.

The Manchester Arena bombing, along with the Westminster attack a few weeks earlier and the London Bridge attack a few weeks later, suggested that our emergency services were involved in a war of sorts on the UK's streets. As such, the public suddenly saw what valuable assets we were. And valuable assets need to be looked after properly.

I've heard that some emergency service staff who attended the Manchester bombing were still off work with PTSD more than a year after the event. Maybe some never returned. It's perhaps not appropriate to talk about silver linings where terrorist attacks are concerned, but they did at least succeed in focusing minds on the vital importance of providing staff with sufficient psychological support, as well as the right knowledge and equipment. My chief executive said to me, 'If it wasn't for the work you were doing prior to this, I don't think we would have delivered support in the way we have.' With another atrocity inevitable, the consensus seemed to be that 999 staff needed to be mentally prepared. The penny seemed to have dropped that support shouldn't just be offered in the wake of an atrocity, it should be on tap. There were lots of meetings, events and bold pronouncements. Change seemed to be afoot.

As part of the NHS's seventieth birthday celebrations, me and Rich received a public tribute and a Points of Light award (which are for outstanding volunteers making a change in their community) from Theresa May (though I couldn't attend 10 Downing Street because I knackered my back the week before). And at the 2018 NHS Heroes Awards in London, me and Rich received the Mental Health Champion honour. In a line-up for the Duchess of Cornwall (Camilla to me and you), I was stood next to Tito Jackson. When everyone was shushing each other and getting giddy about the arrival of Camilla, I was more interested in having a chinwag with Tito about The Jackson 5.

The award was presented to us by the actor Michael Sheen, and there was also a lovely video message from Prince William, who is a former colleague, having been an air ambulance pilot for a couple of years. And as I was stood on the stage, I thought about that policeman who had written me off as a kid, the one who told my head-teacher that I was a bad person and destined to end up in prison. I so hoped he was watching.

Also at the NHS Heroes Awards, I met a girl called Freya Lewis, who survived the Manchester bombing. Freya was only fourteen at the time, and just a few metres away from the explosion. Tragically, her best friend died. Freya was in hospital for six weeks, underwent seventy hours of surgery and had to learn to walk again. But she was back at school just four months after the attack and has raised tens of thousands of pounds for various causes since. Freya was one of the most incredible people I'd ever met, a force of nature. She still has scars, both outside and inside, but she just keeps ploughing on regardless.

Freya confirmed what I already suspected, that there are amazing people out there who are able to turn suffer-ing into something positive. And she made me think of Roger, my wonderful counsellor who had set me on a simi-lar path. I'd always wanted to tell Roger what a positive effect he'd had on me, and so many others by extension. Everything that had happened to me since getting back on my feet, and the changes I'd been able to effect, stemmed from him. But when I next visited my GP surgery with one of my kids, I noticed a book of condolences in the waiting room. Roger had died of cancer, which meant I never got to tell him how much he'd helped me. When you want to say something, don't delay. Otherwise, you might leave it too late.

21

DOING BETTER

You can't see what we see and deal with what we deal with without it having an adverse effect on you. Pretty much every one of my colleagues will have been haunted by difficult memories or nightmares related to the job at some point. I've seen quite a few of them seek solace in alcohol. And I've seen relationships fall apart – including mine.

All the while I was receiving plaudits for raising awareness of mental illness, my marriage was grinding to its end. Our once stable relationship was unable to withstand the collapse of my mental wellbeing. You need the different tracks of your life to run parallel, but my PTSD was like an explosion going off. When that side of the track became bent and tangled, all the weight fell on my marriage. And eventually the marriage couldn't stand the strain and toppled sideways.

It was very difficult for Amy, because I became an arsehole overnight. One minute, I was a loving husband, the next I didn't seem to care less about anything. I'm reassured I was a good father throughout, but I didn't think I was. I didn't think I was attentive enough, but maybe that was related to the guilt of being unwell and thinking that everything I touched turned to dust.

My wife was a better person than me, wanted to talk things through and try to work things out, but I just wanted out of the situation and to focus on my campaigning. The relationship just wasn't for me any more, and I was as blasé as that. Through no fault of her own, I associated Amy with that terrible experience with the murdered child. She was part of the package. I needed a fresh start in life, a total clear-out. So I let the relationship dwindle and die. Me and Amy still have a healthy friendship, and a beautiful boy who is at the centre of everything we do. But I like my new-found freedom.

Of late, I've seen colleagues who started out in the job full of beans crumble before my eyes. It's not just that I'm now better equipped to see the signs, it's just a lot more obvious. The stresses and strains have become so great that some people just aren't able to hide it. Most people can do the job with the right support. But there isn't enough of it.

Even now, a colleague will suddenly disappear and people will say, 'Oh, I hear Joe Bloggs has left.' And someone will reply, 'Yeah, I think he just didn't fancy it any more.' People still don't put two and two together and think that maybe the reason Joe Bloggs 'didn't fancy it any more' was because of the crushing workload and the terrible things he'd seen.

According to the trade union GMB, 81,669 days of sick leave were taken by ambulance staff in England because of mental illness in 2016–18. According to the charity Mind, 91 per cent of ambulance staff have experienced mental health problems as a result of work, a figure that is significantly higher than in the general population. One in four ambulance workers will consider taking their own life at some point in their career, but they are less likely to take time off work or ask for help. I suspect that's partly because of the macho culture – we're supposed to come to the rescue, not the other way around – and the fear that admitting they're struggling will lead colleagues to think they're nuts.

But it's also because ambulance workers don't know who to ask. And when we do ask, there is no clear support structure in place. The culture is changing and more ambulance workers are admitting they're struggling, which is a good and a bad thing: good that they're talking, bad that they're being put under so much pressure that they're having to ask for help.

Another thing counting against ambulance staff is the lack of a single, coherent trade union. Firefighters have the Fire Brigades Union, which most uniformed staff are a member of. Police officers aren't allowed to join a union by law, but they have the Police Federation looking out for their interests. Ambulance staff, however, have several unions, which dilutes our voice. They can be very good at representing you if you're in trouble but when it comes to pay or the retirement age, they can be a bit weak.

When you're at the bargaining table with politicians, you're far better off being represented by one booming voice, rather than a lot of shrill ones all arguing with each other. I'm not a militant man and would never dream of going on strike. How could I when it would mean people dying? But I would like a strong body that stands up for its staff. And part of standing up for your staff is making sure they have sufficient health and wellbeing provision.

While the ambulance service might blame a lack of resources and time for the deficiency in its mental health provision, there are solutions to every problem. If they have to be cost-effective, then make them cost-effective. They have to want to find solutions, and they have a responsibility to find solutions. But the only people who can make them live up to that responsibility are politicians.

In an ideal world, the HR department would say, 'If we invest in the wellbeing of our staff, we will save money in sick leave and retention.' But that's long-term thinking, and ambulance service bosses, in common with bosses in all the emergency services, already have enough on their plates plugging holes, baling out water and keeping their respective ships afloat.

The government has suggested that every workplace should have a mental health first aider. That's great, but mental health first aid is like a sticking plaster. Ambulance people see and deal with terrible things on a weekly basis, so what works for an average work environment is unlikely to be sufficient for the ambulance service. What comes before physical first aid in the workplace? A robust health and safety policy, so that people don't fall down stairs and off ladders in the first place. In the same way, mental health first aid should be superseded by a robust mental health and wellbeing policy.

Like any workers, ambulance staff have yearly appraisals. But those appraisals are focused on the actual work, along with targets, box-ticking and form-filling. That's all well and good, but appraisals should also be like spring cleans for employees' minds, or mental MOTs, a root around under an employee's bonnet to see if everything is working as it should be. If you owned a factory full of machines, you'd spend money making sure those machines were maintained. Because if they weren't maintained, they would inevitably go wrong, not perform their jobs properly and your business would suffer.

Frontline ambulance staff should be taught resilience building, or how best to cope with the stresses of the job. Resilience is a life skill, and it shouldn't just be taught to ambulance staff, it should be taught to people working in every emergency service. In fact, it should be taught to everyone, including kids in schools.

Many people don't even have a concept of what mental health is, let alone how to maintain it. I gave a talk once, during which I said, 'How many people in this room have mental health?' A couple of hands went up. Then I said, 'Actually, everyone in this room has mental health, just as we all have physical health. It's one of the things that makes us human. And as long as you have mental health, you're at risk of developing a mental health problem.' There were one or two confused faces, but when I told my story, they understood the point I was making: only when you fully understand yourself and the potential problems you might face can you know when to seek help.

People need to know how to recognise when they are okay and when they're not. Your relationship might be misfunctioning. Your child might be unwell. You might be struggling financially. You might be struggling to sleep. You might be drinking too much and eating too much rubbish. Things add up, compact in your mind, and that one final straw might send you crashing through the floor.

Some people don't like the idea of speaking to a psychiatrist or counsellor, but they might like talking about work with their colleagues, whether it's bitching about bosses or politics or the quality of the coffee in the vending machine. However banal those conversations might sound to people outside the group, they are important to those in it, because work plays such a big part in people's lives. You become part of a brother- and sisterhood in the ambulance service, no different to being in the police force or the military. As such, I'm a big believer in using peer support to tackle mental health issues.

There should be colleagues, whether current or former members of frontline ambulance staff, who people can talk to in a controlled environment, in absolute confidence. Some emergency services have introduced a tool called TRiM (Trauma Risk Management), which was born in the military in the 1990s. TRiM is about teaching people to assess colleagues' responses to a specific traumatic event. If someone has dealt with something potentially traumatic, they can talk to a TRiM assessor (who is a colleague, not a medical professional), who is trained to identify whether they might need to be referred for counselling.

TRiM is a good idea in theory, except ambulance workers don't work on the frontline of a warzone (not technically, anyway), where the provision of on-the-spot counselling is naturally less practical. We should be able to speak to professionals whenever we need to, not have to rely on the well-meaning guesswork of colleagues. Some services do have counsellors you can call free of charge, but often this involves a few weeks' wait to speak to somebody.

I like to use the analogy of a building site. Until fairly recently, health and safety on building sites was negligible. It was common to see labourers working without hard hats well into the 1980s. Someone wearing ear defenders and a high-vis jacket would have been a total laughing stock. But back in 1974, the government passed the Health and Safety at Work Act. It didn't improve the situation immediately, but accidents and deaths reduced slowly but surely.

In 1981, the fatality rate for construction workers was 7.9 per 100,000 – four times higher than the rate across the general workforce. In 2016, it was 1.9 per 100,000. Now there is barely a building site in the country that doesn't adhere to the health and safety rules and regulations, and any boss of a construction company who is caught flouting health and safety rules and regulations is seen as a cowboy at best and a criminal at worst.

My hope is that at some point in the near future, we'll look back at the ambulance service's mental health provision and be appalled at how inadequate it was. Sending staff out to deal with traumatic situations without providing sufficient support is every bit as negligent as allowing people to climb ladders minus hard hats and without anyone holding the bottom.

The situation isn't all doom and gloom. Ambulance people are a band of brothers and sisters and we try to look out for each other. But we can all do better. We don't engage our instincts and listen for signs. We walk into a room and say, 'Morning. You okay?' And most people will reply, 'Yeah, all good, mate', or something along those lines. But someone might say, 'No, I've had a bit of a shit morning actually.' That person might be trying to tell you something. They might be tentatively reaching out for help, which might only consist of a chat. But too often when we ask someone if they're okay, we don't listen to their answer. And the uncomfortable truth is, too many people roll their eyes and think, *What a miserable sod*.

And I'm not just talking about the ambulance service. The same can be said for most work and social environments. I've heard professional footballers talk about wanting to cry in the dressing room before a game, while knowing they'll be mocked if they show as much as a flicker of emotion. But if you notice even the smallest of signs – a friend being unusually quiet or irritable, falling out of love with former interests, expressing negative thoughts – maybe ask if everything is okay. And if they say yes, ask them again.

22

ANOTHER WAY

In 2018, I was awarded a Churchill Fellowship to research
mental health and wellbeing in the American and
Canadian emergency services. Fellows are given a grant
by the Winston Churchill Memorial Trust and sent off to
learn how people in other countries deal with issues we
have encountered in our lives. It's a brilliantly simple idea,
empowering people to learn from the world for the benefit
of the UK.

I already knew from my research that people in America
and Canada had done extensive work in the field and had
world-class support structures in place. So I was tremendously excited about what ideas I might bring home with
me. I felt like a Victorian explorer setting off for an exotic
land with a butterfly net.

First stop was New York and the 9/11 Memorial & Museum. I couldn't even begin to imagine what the city's first responders went through the day the World Trade Center came crashing down, but the museum does a very good job of telling their story. Clearly, one of the museum's aims was to ensure those emergency workers and the people they tried to save would never be forgotten, which made me think about how the UK's emergency workers are viewed. America is very good at lionising those who put their lives and wellbeing on the line for their country, whether it be their soldiers, firefighters or ambulance workers. The UK, not so much. Too often, the police are portrayed as prejudiced and bent and firefighters as lazy. Ambulance workers might as well be invisible.

I spent a week with the Las Vegas Metropolitan Police Department, leading up to the first anniversary of the Mandalay Bay massacre, in which fifty-eight people were killed. I wanted to see how they had supported their staff in the wake of the shooting, and what I found out amazed me. They had a whole department of former police officers whose job was to provide non-judgemental mental health peer support. These were people who knew what it was to be on the frontline and had received tailored training, rather than counsellors who could only guess. They were housed in a secluded, non-descript building away from the police station, so that an officer in need wouldn't feel nervous about being seen entering. This peer support department also provided a pathway for older members of staff who otherwise might have retired and ended up feeling bereft and forgotten by the service.

Any Las Vegas police officer involved in a fatal shooting has to be referred to a counsellor, with the recommendation that that relationship be maintained for at least six months. When they offered to show me the board with the names of coppers who'd shot people and were receiving treatment, I expected there to be two or three. In fact, the whole board was covered. While it was shocking to see just how prevalent gun deaths are in America, it was also heart-warming to know that all those people were being unconditionally supported. Also on the menu was musculoskeletal treatment and a range of alternative therapies. It made health and wellbeing provision in the UK ambulance service look medieval.

At Louisiana State University in Baton Rouge, they were doing amazing things to support their students' mental health, which I thought could be applied to people doing paramedic degrees in the UK. There was a lot of emphasis on building resilience, including the importance of leading a healthy lifestyle, exercising, eating well and looking after your finances. And what struck me most about their support network was its openness. If a student had a problem of any description, whether it be a drink, drugs or gambling addiction, they were safe in the knowledge that they could reach out for help without being judged or censured.

In New Orleans, I looked at a few more left-field treatments, such as music therapy and even beer yoga. Supping on a beer while in the downward dog position was surprisingly relaxing, although I'm not sure the bosses back home would be sold on the idea. New Orleans was a real eye-opener in terms of the level of crime their emergency services have to deal with. I spent a few hours with a New Orleans police officer, and that day he'd been to an armed robbery at a petrol station in which the man behind the till was shot dead at point blank range, and a drive-by shooting which left three people dead and a ten-year-old injured. That's probably the same number of murders I've dealt with in fifteen years working for the ambulance service in the UK.

I was blown away by the ambulance services up in Canada. In Ottawa, they have a great peer support network, but arguably more important than that, mental health support is written into law. So instead of *asking* the emergency services to improve mental health provision for their staff, the authorities *told* them they *had* to. That's a big difference, because you can put all the pretty pleases in the world at the end of a request and it can still be ignored. But if you write something into law and make it part of management's targets, they will jump to attention. Managers in Canada not having a choice meant their workplace policies were a country mile ahead of ours.

Ambulance workers in Ottawa had the very best vehicles, the very best kit, the very best equipment and the very best uniforms. Everything seemed to be bang on. They also had 'make-ready teams', whose job was to prepare each ambulance before it went out for a shift. All the paramedics had to do was turn up, grab the keys and go, without having to worry if anyone had nicked a cylinder of Entonox from the back.

They also employed a traffic light self-assessment tool to encourage staff to talk about any mental health issues. You turn up at work and someone will say, 'Are you in your green today?' If the answer is no, you're feeling amber, then it might be time to have a chinwag with someone, even if the issue isn't directly related to work. If you're in the red, it's definitely time for a chinwag. It might sound a bit corny to a cynical British readership, but the overriding feedback from the rank and file staff was that they felt valued. And there is an understanding from bosses that if you value your staff, you will reduce sickness, increase retention and make working for the ambulance service feel less thankless.

Not that the nitty-gritty of the job was much different. Riding in an Ottawa ambulance as an observer, the first job we went to was an attempted suicide. A woman just out of the army and struggling to come to terms with civilian life had driven her car into a lamp post. When we got back to the station at the end of the shift, there were staff there who had just been to another traumatic incident. No one was talking, a couple of them were teary. And then a therapy dog came bouncing in, acting daft as a brush. Everyone was stroking and cuddling it, and suddenly the same people who had been silent and crying were laughing and chatting about the job they'd just been to. It was miraculous. The dog even went out to jobs in an ambulance car. I understand there are businesses trialling therapy dogs in the UK. And they work – I've seen it! – and are testament to the benefits of thinking outside the box.

In Maryland, I spent time with the Bladensburg Fire Department. Bladensburg is a little bit rough around the edges and most famous for an 1812 battle in which the British routed the Americans, but the locals didn't seem to mind me being there. On my first morning, I was having a nice cup of coffee in the station when the hooter went off. Me and the lads piled into the engine and we tear-arsed towards a house fire. There was no holding back, they went straight into this burning wooden building with their hose pipe and seemingly no regard for their own safety.

A few minutes later, another engine turned up from another station, and I couldn't help picking up on a bit of animosity between the two crews. It was only afterwards I learned that both sets of crews were volunteers, and there was something close to a sporting rivalry between them. That's not ideal, but what I learned from the Bladensburg lads was the benefit of an emergency service operating as a tightknit team. They were a community, a family. And they loved their job, even though they weren't even being paid for putting their lives at risk. There were no formal support networks in place, they just had each other. It confirmed my belief that mental health provision isn't just the responsibility of employers, it's the responsibility of all of us.

I wasn't a fan of their leather helmets, though. One bloke got hit on the head by a piece of wood and a nail went into his face. I said to him afterwards, 'Why don't you get some decent lids?' He replied, 'We've had these for years, we'd never change them.' It just goes to show that workers all over the world can get stuck in their ways and you will always find things that can be done better.

In Paramus, New Jersey, I spent time with two lovely ladies who had set up something called the Paramus Stigma-Free Zone. Their aim is a grand one: to build a society in which people are free of the stigma of mental illness and can access the help they need without fear of being judged. They put up signs in schools, offices and first responder stations, declaring them stigma-free zones. Anyone can sign up, and a lot of people have.

When you sign up, you have to pledge to do something to reduce the stigma of mental illness. That might be organising a stigma-free football game or barbeque – or any event where people can gather and feel comfortable talking about their mental wellbeing. It's about giving people the tools to be able to discuss mental health and change the way society views it. They loved the fact that I was this guy who had travelled all the way from England to learn from them. That, in a nutshell, is what a Churchill Fellowship is all about.

Stigma-free zones will feature prominently in my fellowship report. But aside from my report, I need advocates in Parliament. You would think a pledge to look after 999 workers better would be a vote winner, but at the moment workplace wellbeing isn't even on Parliament's agenda. Finding politicians to push my recommendations is the easy part. Finding politicians who are genuinely passionate about the issue might be more difficult. I also need to gather more empirical evidence. If I can say to the powers that be, 'By investing x amount of money in each ambulance worker's wellbeing, you will save x amount of money further down the line, by reducing sick leave and increasing retention,' then I'll have their attention. Appealing to the emotions of these people is one thing; you need to waft cold, hard numbers under their noses to get them to take action.

I'd love the fellowship paper to lead to legislative change and I'm always hopeful. Perfect legislation would include resilience training before we even start out on the road, a clear referral pathway, regular mental health 'MOTs' and mental health professionals with an intimate knowledge of the problems faced by ambulance workers, on tap. Weaved into that would be a directive for bosses to implement visible peer-led grassroots support. I'd also like guaranteed funding for the NHS to enable all this to happen. But never mind money, it needs to happen because it's the right thing to happen.

23

SOFTENING THE BLOW

Recently, I moved to a different area within the same service. I fancied somewhere a bit more rural, away from the smoke. And, just maybe, with a bit less stress. After my final shift working out of my old station, I parked up the ambulance, hung up the keys and went home. That was that.

Ambulance people are defined by the work they do. But one day you're Joe Bloggs the paramedic, the next you're out of the service and no longer that person. Who are you now? Where does life take you from there? I call it career bereavement. And often when ambulance workers retire, they're suddenly stuck in an armchair all day, mulling over twenty or thirty years of trauma, with no one to talk to and all the horrible stuff they've dealt with swirling around their heads.

A few of my retired colleagues have come to me for help, including one chap who had moved abroad and I assumed was enjoying his retirement in the sun. One day, he phoned me in tears. He told me about his nightmares and that he felt betrayed by the ambulance service. He was one of the loveliest, most respected guys I'd ever worked with, and he thought he'd been part of this special organisation, something like a family. But when he retired, he realised he was just a counter in a game, swept off the board and forgotten. That might be fine if you worked in an office for thirty years, but not if you've been exposed to the things he was exposed to in the course of his career.

I spent a few hours on the phone to him and we've kept in contact since. I send him snippets of gossip from the station, so that he feels like he's still part of the gang. I hope he takes some comfort from that. But the ambulance service shouldn't be allowing people to feel neglected. This guy gained his mental scars serving his country with the ambulance service for decades, so why is the ambulance service not supporting him in his retirement?

Recently, the manager who suggested a job on the front-line of the ambulance service might not be for me took me aside and said, 'I was wrong, you've opened my eyes.'

But another manager told me that by raising awareness of mental illness, I was creating problems. He thought my campaigning was counter-productive, because it was making staff question themselves. I understood his point. There is a fine line. Can you offer too much support, so that people who don't have a problem convince themselves they do have a problem? Maybe you can be too insistent:

'Are you okay?'

'Yes, I'm fine.'

'Are you absolutely sure you're okay?'

'Yes! Stop mithering me about it!'

Maybe there is something to be said for being stoic and plodding along, like in the old days. And maybe there are psychiatrists who would say that some things are best left buried. But it's not something I was able to do.

There are colleagues who haven't spoken to me since I went down with PTSD and started talking about it. Maybe they think that mental illness is something that shouldn't be discussed. Maybe they think I'm a loon. There were certainly people who thought I was milking the situation and enjoying the limelight a bit too much. One colleague said to me, 'I've been in this job twenty-five years and I've never been given opportunities like you have.' I replied, 'It's not about me getting to meet the royal family. It's about highlighting the lack of support for mental illness in the service – the service you work for! It's about the thousands of people we've been able to reach and help.'

If there are a couple of people who think I'm milking my PTSD and what I'm trying to achieve is a waste of time, I can live with that. Most people love what we're doing; the naysayers are few and far between. The stigma of mental illness is being reduced on the shop floor, in that people are generally more accepting and open about the subject. We've got people talking, which is great. Senior managers and politicians have to take recommendations on board and join the discussion. Only then will major legislative changes be made. But it's going to take time for that attitude to work its way up the food chain.

When I first started campaigning, the bosses really got on board with it. But as soon as Mind wound up their Blue Light Programme and my work with the royal family tailed off, so did the ambulance service's enthusiasm. A phone number for a counsellor pinned to a notice board is not nearly enough.

An attempt to set up a network of emergency services across the whole of my region, so that they could share knowledge, also foundered. The hope was that if one service created something that worked, they could share their idea with the others. A few of the services who really wanted to improve their mental health provision bought into it, but not everyone shared their enthusiasm. It was disappointing, but I wasn't surprised. I guess it's something that still makes some people feel uncomfortable.

Indifference and scepticism are sometimes difficult to deal with. But – and this is a sentence I thought I'd never write – I found that poetry helped. While I was in America, I attended a couple of poetry readings in bars and discovered 'If' by Rudyard Kipling. It seemed like a good lesson in how to be a genuine person, which is what I was striving to be. Every now and again, when I'm feeling a bit unsure of myself or the direction I've taken, I'll pull it up on my phone and reread it. There are certainly a few lines in there that any ambulance person can relate to, not least, 'If you can trust yourself when all men doubt you, But make allowance for their doubting too.'

———

I've not become immune to the things I see, but I've become more hardened to them. They call that post traumatic resilience and growth. Being laid low by PTSD was a horrible time in my life, and sometimes when I think about what happened it scares me. But the crumbling brickwork that undermined me has been cemented solid. I'm no longer having counselling and I feel a lot more robust and able to deal with the trauma I'm exposed to. And it's made me a better person. I'm more aware of my feelings and the feelings of people around me, and I draw strength from helping people through difficult times, whether they be current or former colleagues, people from other emergency services or other walks of life completely.

The story about the seven-week-old baby at the beginning of this book happened fairly recently. It is yet more proof that you never get used to dealing with jobs as harrowing as that. But you can learn how to soften the blow. After trying and failing to save that baby, I filled out the necessary paperwork before talking to the doctors and nurses in A&E. I found that therapeutic, and I think they did, too. Back at the station, I discussed it with my colleagues. They were genuinely interested from a technical point of view, because they wondered what they would have done in the same situation. I took a lot of comfort from just chewing the fat. Before my downfall, I might not have even mentioned it.

I made sure to tell my partner on the job, who was fairly new and had never dealt with anything as harrowing, that she didn't have to bottle up what she'd seen, that she could have a chat with me any time and that there were other people who could help. I was also able to tell her that, despite being laid low by the things I'd seen in the past, I was still doing the very best I could.

I hadn't slept for twenty-four hours, so you'd think I'd have staggered through my front door and crashed out on the sofa. Instead, I stared at the ceiling, haunted by the screams and laments of the baby's parents. And when I finally drifted off, I had a nightmare, in which I saw the baby dying all over again. I can still see that baby now, even when I'm wide awake. I doubt I'll ever forget her face. But now I feel strong enough to deal with the memory.

24

TREMENDOUSLY PROUD

I've had a strange life in some ways. Certainly, some strange stuff has happened to me. Then again, I don't think any ambulance person would say any different. But I wouldn't change a thing, because I've also had some incredible opportunities. I've had a ringside seat for the very best and the very worst of humanity. I've witnessed humbling kindness and breath-taking depravity. I've dealt with wonderful people I've forgotten and awful people I can't erase from my memory. And having been floored by the job and bounced off the deck still punching, I feel like it's my responsibility to inspire people.

Hopefully, people will read this book and realise that mental illness doesn't have to define you, that you can still lead a worthwhile and fulfilling life. Despite what happened to me, I'm still cracking on with things, raising my kids and managing to do a challenging job to a high standard, day in, day out.

I've been let down a lot in my life. But one of the biggest let-downs was how I felt I was treated by my employers when I was struggling with the stresses of the job. I don't want that to happen to anyone else. I've always been fuelled by injustice, and an ambulance service without proper mental health and wellbeing provision is not a just ambulance service. But if changes are made, future generations of ambulance workers – and workers in general – will feel safer and more valued in the workplace. That's why I'd love to set up a service that offers health and wellbeing solutions to companies. I'd go in and give resilience training to staff. Make sure they know when they're well and when they're not. Explain to them that everyone is susceptible to mental illness, that there is nothing to be gained from hiding problems and no shame in asking for help.

I've managed to get people talking, but that's just the first step. Charitable campaigns come and go. Mind's Blue Light Programme was funded by Libor fines, but that funding was pulled in 2018. As a result, there is no longer targeted funding for mental health awareness in the emergency services. But there are still some good charities doing sterling work and a lot of different people looking into the problem. And I'm more determined than ever to persuade the powers that be to act. I won't stop until mental health and workplace wellbeing is treated as seriously as it should be. PTSD couldn't beat me, so I won't let a little thing like Parliament get in my way.

I try to practise what I preach. After the incident with the seven-week-old baby, and despite my harrowing nightmare, I didn't feel the need to see a professional counsellor. Because I'd already been through similar, I was more resilient and able to self-assess. I talked it over with colleagues and drew strength from their empathy. That was enough for me, although it might not be enough for everyone.

I phone my mum on the way home from work every single day. She and my dad have been with me every step of the way, including through my struggles with PTSD. Mum's my safe person, someone to offload on, no different to a counsellor. I mainly talk and she mainly listens. It makes perfect sense, but how many people do the same? My mum and dad were instrumental in making my four kids the amazing people they are, having pulled out all the stops when things went wrong for me. I don't know what I would have been without their help. As it is, my kids are also my four best friends and mean absolutely everything to me. Now, all I aspire to be in life is the best parent I can possibly be.

I've seen some horrendous things, but my mind is capable of conjuring even worse. I had another nightmare recently in which I was sent to a major incident. When I arrived on the scene, I found a load of my colleagues lying dead. A psychologist would have a field day with that one. It was a horrible vision and I woke up soaked through with sweat. But it's possible the nightmare had a positive message: what's the worst thing that can happen if you get ill or have an accident? That there will be nobody there to help you. That tells you how incredibly important ambulance workers are to society.

My brief appearance atop *Heat* magazine's Manometer aside, ambulance workers don't have the sexiest of images among the public. Teenage girls do not have posters on their wall of paramedics stripped to the waist, as they might of a firefighter. Authors do not write books about fictional ambulance workers, and directors rarely make films about the ambulance service, as they often do about the police force. And sometimes when I tell people I'm an ambulance person, they give me a look that says, 'Why would anyone want to do that?'

I sometimes say I became an ambulance person by accident. But it can't have been that much of an accident, because I'm still doing the job fifteen years later. And I do the job because I want to. The hours and workload are trying, rendering us permanently weary and often stressed. We see things that make us question humanity. And when we think we've seen it all – which is a common occurrence – something will happen that makes us realise we probably never will. The work can transform people into emotional wrecks or make them cold and detached, and neither is ideal. The pay is decidedly average and we often feel underappreciated, neglected and disrespected. Sometimes we get punched. Sometimes we get spat at. But most people seem to understand that we're only trying to help.

It's easy to become cynical about the ambulance service and the NHS in general when you're exposed to their inner workings. But when the public needs us, and despite the glitches, we usually come up trumps. I will never forget the people who came to my rescue when I was stabbed and my twins were in special care. Their desperation to make things better was palpable. And most people will have similar stories about the ambulance service.

We're there when you're a baby and running a wicked fever, when you fall out of a tree and break your arm, when you drink too much and pass out, when you crash your car, when you're having a heart attack, when you fall over in the garden, when you can't get out of bed, when you're nearing the end and you want someone to help you die in a dignified manner.

I'm tremendously proud to say I work for the ambulance service and I have a deep love for the job. It might not be the sexiest occupation, but it's one of the most rewarding.

How many people can say they arrived home late from work or missed their child's sports day because they were saving someone's life? Or making someone's last moments on earth as comfortable as possible? Or listening to the first cries and splutters of a newborn baby? How many people can say they really make a difference? I care passionately about the people I treat. I've had moments when I've thought, *Do I really need this?* But then I think, *Even if I don't need this job, the people I treat need me.*

We start out in the job wide-eyed and idealistic, thinking we can save every patient we deal with. That naivety soon gives way to narrow-eyed cynicism and the harsh realisation that some patients are simply beyond help. In some ways, medical professionals are like professional sportspeople. The things they remember most vividly are the things that go wrong. For a footballer, it might be missing a penalty or being sent off in a cup final. For an ambulance person, it might be a murdered child dying in their arms. And, in common with a lot of boxers, an ambulance person's work can take more than it gives and leave them feeling punch-drunk and gun-shy.

It makes me sad when I hear people say, 'I've got no sympathy for the ambulance service' – maybe because they had to wait for hours for an ambulance to turn up while a loved one was writhing in pain. It's nothing personal and, 99.9 per cent of the time, ambulance staff aren't responsible for turning up late. I'd like people to know what a great set of people ambulance workers are and that despite everything they're up against, they're doing a wonderful job. There is no typical frontline ambulance person. They come from all different walks of life, which makes it a diverse, exciting workforce. But they all share one thing in common: a love for their patients, a love for their colleagues and a love for the job.

Ambulance workers tend to be very stoic and very humble. They don't do the job for praise. They do it because they want to help people. A problem with humble people is that they are easy to ignore, take for granted and take advantage of. I feel huge loyalty to the public and my colleagues. And not just my colleagues in the ambulance service, but also in other parts of the NHS, the fire service, prison service and police force – or indeed any public servant who is doing a difficult job in incredibly trying circumstances. Writing this book was the best present I could give them. I hope my colleagues will read it and say, 'Thank God someone else has spoken up about the problems we face.'

Ambulance people are doing the best they can with what they've got, which is never enough. And it's import-ant to remember that the ambulance service isn't just made up of paramedics, technicians and EMDs. There are also mechanics, IT people, telecommunications people, cleaners, people who do the rotas, people who purchase our equipment. Remove one of these branches and the whole ambulance service would come crashing down.

I also hope that people might now understand that when an ambulance person says they're fine, they might not be fine at all. If you have a mate working in the ambulance or emergency services or the NHS, maybe phone them up and ask them how they are. And don't take 'fine' for an answer.

As for me, things are marginally less stressful on my new patch in the sticks. I'm also studying to become a paramedic, rather than a technician. But will I work for the ambulance service for ever? No, because I know that when I'm sixty-seven, I won't be able to provide the service my patients deserve. Sometimes I think I'd like to go back and work in a garden centre. No real responsibilities, just chinwagging with people about plant pots and geraniums. Dig the fish net out every now and again and chase a carp around the pond. That'll do me.

But when I do hang up my keys in the station for the last time, I'll miss the job and the sheer thrill of helping people like hell. It's a tough gig, but someone has to do it. And I'm glad it's me. I feel like the luckiest man in the world.

25

TAKING ON CORONAVIRUS

If I were a more superstitious man, I'd claim I was responsible for coronavirus. Here's why. It's New Year's Eve and I'm out in the ambulance with one of my managers. He's a funny lad, a bit of a legend. It's coming up to midnight, so we grab a cup of coffee from the hospital and head back to the station.

We do the awkward countdown, cheers each other with coffee cups and have a little bet on when the first call of 2020 will be. Just for the laugh, no money involved. I say 12.10, my mate says 12.07. We both reason that once everyone's had a hug and a singsong, people will soon start hitting each other and falling over. The first call comes in at about 12.09. I've won the bet. Then I make the mistake of saying, 'Tell you what, pal, this job will define the rest of the year.' My mate replies, 'Don't say that. This job could be a pile of rubbish.'

Our first patient of 2020 has a lot of problems going on but has fallen through the cracks, like so many others. She's known to be violent, so we hover around the corner from her house, making small talk, while waiting for the police. When the police arrive, we follow them in and find this lady in her bedroom. She hasn't self-harmed, but she is saying she feels suicidal, so we need to take her to hospital. But upon leaving the house, she suddenly becomes aggressive, so we step away and let the police do their thing. They manage to calm her down and get her into the back of the ambulance, at which point she gets very agitated and spits straight in my face. Happy new year.

I freeze. I don't know how to react. Eventually, I step off the ambulance and try to gather my thoughts, while the police are bundling her into the back of their van. I feel dirty and humiliated. All I want to do is get back home and have a shower. Not much is said on the journey back to the station, until my mate says, 'Well, at least you've learned a lesson tonight. Because of you and your big mouth, that woman has defined our year.' A few months later, every NHS employee was living in fear of being spat at, deliberately or otherwise. It wasn't just a horrible thing to happen, it was something that could kill you.

The coronavirus pandemic came crashing into the

NHS from seemingly nowhere. When the media started reporting on this strange disease spreading like wildfire in China, I didn't take much notice. I'd heard it all before, whether it was SARS, swine flu or Ebola. What usually happens is the media work the public into a panic and the disease never actually arrives.

There had been a lot of people ill at Christmas, including in my own family, but people are always ill at Christmas. When a nurse told me that a Chinese tourist had presented herself at hospital with a bad cough and cold and asked for a test, the staff didn't know what she meant. They told her to go home and drink a Lemsip, probably cursing her for wasting time, albeit in their heads.

Even when the media started reporting on cases in the UK, I heard colleagues saying, 'It's nothing to worry about. It can't be much worse than flu.' And then it got serious, as if someone had flicked a switch. In early March, I was sent to a couple who had returned home from Cyprus, both incredibly unwell, short of breath and with temperatures through the roof. The wife was confused, didn't know what day of the week it was. That was the first time I thought, 'Hmmm, this looks like this coronavirus they've been telling us about.' We informed the hospital, but they still weren't sure. At that point, most people thought coronavirus was something that only came out of China.

Within a couple of weeks, we were wearing Tyvek

suits and respirators. That didn't last long. Once it started spreading, for the majority of call-outs they ditched the *CSI: Miami* gear and had us wearing pinnies, masks and gloves instead. One extreme to the next. Presumably they started out by thinking it wasn't going to be too bad, before realising it was going to be very bad indeed and there wasn't enough *CSI: Miami* gear to go round. After that, the rules around Personal Protective Equipment (PPE) – when to wear it, when not to wear it – kept changing, almost on a daily basis.

Paramedics are very adaptable, but it was difficult to keep up with what we were supposed to be doing. There was nothing on my training course about pandemics. Rooms at the station were limited to a certain amount of people, and chairs were rearranged to encourage social distancing. We had to wear a mask pretty much 12 hours a day: at the station, in the ambulance on the way to a job, in patients' houses. Colleagues' glasses would fog up. The wind would blow the pinny in your face as soon as you stepped off the ambulance. They sound like small things, but they made hard jobs even more difficult.

Any aerosol-generated procedures, such as treating a cardiac arrest, became extremely challenging. That's when we'd have to stick the whole nine yards on: goggles, visor, Tyvek suit, which would stop fluid getting in but also stop fluid getting out, so that it was like roasting in an oven.

It didn't help that spring was so warm and summer came early. Doing CPR and trying to cannulate and intubate people became very difficult. There was sweat pouring down my forehead and into my eyes, so that I couldn't see what I was doing. It showed just how out of shape I was, but I did lose a few pounds. Every cloud.

A smile can fix a lot of things. It's a paramedic's trustiest bit of kit. It can put a patient at ease, give them hope and a lot more besides. But coronavirus meant smiles were cancelled indefinitely. I'd still be cracking them out, it's just that patients wouldn't be able to see them behind my mask. It didn't help that a lot of the older boys and girls were unable to make out what we were saying, because they were hard of hearing and usually relied on watching people's lips.

Some of the miscommunications were like a *Two Ronnies* sketch. One day, we went out to two chaps, one of whom was complaining of constipation. Not really the sort of thing you should be calling 999 for. They were both drunk and quite angry and we couldn't get much sense out of them. The fact that they were wearing masks, as well as us, made communicating almost impossible.

One of the first things the patient said to me when we walked in was 'John Tennant'. At least that's what I thought he said, which is why I kept calling him John throughout the assessment: 'Everything's going to be all right, John. I'm going to need you to do this, John. I'm now going to do this, John.' But when it came to filling out the forms and I asked him to confirm that his name was indeed John Tennant, he replied, 'My name's Sean. I said we were joint tenants.' I have no idea why he felt the need to tell me that. I can only imagine that he didn't want us to think they were in a romantic relationship.

Once the death toll started rising, NHS workers started getting a bit fearful. I wouldn't call it panic, but people were quite tense and apprehensive. We didn't know what we were getting ourselves into. We didn't know how coronavirus was transferred or what we needed to do to prevent ourselves from getting it. There was a lot of fearmongering, especially on social media. In the early days, people thought that anyone who got it ended up in intensive care. And when people started panic-buying toilet roll, you knew things had got serious. That was just so surreal. For a few mad weeks, nurses and doctors were finishing shifts and not being able to buy basic provisions. I'd never seen selfishness like it. It made me wonder what might have been different, had a pandemic struck before the internet. I think there is a danger of knowing too much, a lot of it nonsense, and I suspect the response might have been more measured.

I started thinking about all the people I'd treated with coronavirus symptoms, like bad chest infections, before it started making the news. I also wondered about all those times I'd sat in the back of the ambulance with people who almost definitely had coronavirus. It's not like we could self-isolate, otherwise the NHS would have fallen apart. Then, from nowhere, I developed a tickly cough, which soon got far worse, combined with a furious temperature. When I phoned work, they told me to stay home for two weeks. I didn't need telling twice. I went straight to my holiday home, so as not to be in contact with my kids. But it wasn't much of a holiday. I'd never felt lethargy like it. I slept for almost two weeks solid and barely ate. I still don't know if I was suffering from coronavirus because there was no testing at the time. I'm convinced it was, because the symptoms were bang on, but I'll probably never find out.

The vast majority of people behaved themselves during lockdown and followed the rules. But there are always exceptions. One day, we were called to a house by the police and told that someone was unconscious. When we arrived, there were four people inside, all from different households. There was lots of beer being drunk and weed being smoked, but none of them was unconscious. While we were telling them that people weren't supposed to be having gatherings, we heard a bang coming from the direction of a wardrobe. When we opened the door, there was a woman inside, who just toppled over. She'd been hiding because she had a history of brawling with one of the men and wasn't supposed to be anywhere near him. A neighbour had grassed them up to get the gathering dispersed, but other than telling everyone to go home, there wasn't much the police could do. You can't manage stupid.

But coronavirus wasn't the nightmare for me that it was for a lot of other NHS workers, because I wasn't dealing with a lot of the stuff I normally deal with. Suddenly, there were no pub brawls or people falling over drunk in the street, banging their heads and breaking bones. Because people weren't driving anywhere, there were fewer road traffic accidents. There were fewer people going for walks and injuring themselves. The commute to work was an absolute dream, because there were hardly any cars on the road. Less good was the fact that people with chest pains and other possible medical emergencies weren't calling 999 because they didn't want to be anywhere near a hospital. At one point, the NHS had to put a message out, reminding people that A&Es were still open for people suffering with things other than coronavirus. And it did reach the stage, at the pandemic's peak in April, when the hospitals looked like they might become overwhelmed. They never did, but the idea that they might made a lot of NHS workers very apprehensive.

———

A call comes in: 16-YEAR-OLD. POSSIBLE HANGING. I put my foot down, reach the address in no time, get all the gear on and pile straight in. But when we get to the top of the stairs and push the door open, we're greeted by the world's biggest Alsatian. I can hear a man in the background, it sounds like he's administering CPR. So I shout, 'Mate, you need to put your dog away!' The guy replies, 'The dog's friendly, just come in!'

We edge our way down the hallway with extreme caution, because we're not convinced this dog is as friendly as the guy claims. But thank God for that dog, because suddenly a girl comes flying out of nowhere brandishing a six-inch knife. Had we gone in any quicker, things might have been very different. I realise that the guy hadn't been doing CPR, he'd actually been trying to restrain this girl. Turns out that she'd tried to tie a rope around her neck and when he'd tried to stop her, she'd grabbed a knife and tried to slash herself. When we turned up, she decided to turn the knife on us instead.

This isn't the first time I've been attacked with a knife. What do you do in that situation? Me and my partner use our bags as shields before the guy manages to hold her down. I run to the ambulance and press the tits-up button. But as trusty as that button is, it has one downside, namely that everything you say is broadcast to everyone on that frequency. And what I say on this occasion is, 'Let's leg it!'

In the background, my partner is still telling the girl to put the knife down.

The police turn up in no time, get the knife off this girl and whisk her to hospital for a mental health evaluation. I give a statement and hear nothing more about her. But I can't get her off my mind. It takes me a long time to calm down and I'm not afraid to say it sets me back quite a bit. I keep thinking, 'If this is what the job is going to be like, maybe it's not for me anymore. I love helping people, but do I really want to do it if it means risking my own life?'

I keep telling myself that she was mentally unwell and didn't know what she was doing, but that didn't make it any less scary. But after a lot of reflecting, I start to think more rationally. In my 16 years on the road, I've been assaulted – punched, spat at, attacked with a knife – maybe once every thousand jobs. And I finally conclude that the benefits of helping people far outweigh the risks. It's not time to hang up my defibrillator just yet.

During the pandemic, paramedics were more valuable than ever, not just for our medical skills, but also for our bedside manner. Visitors not being allowed into hospitals must have been devastating for patients. I'm a 34-year-old man and I'd still want my mum with me if I was ever admitted with something serious. I understood why the measures were introduced, but that didn't make it any easier having to tell people their relatives weren't allowed to accompany them to hospital or see them once they were admitted.

It was heartbreaking to witness. All they wanted was for a relative or friend – someone with a familiar face, a familiar voice, a familiar touch – to hold their hand. Instead, they were surrounded by strange NHS workers wearing masks and protective gear. Those workers were doing their very best, but being in hospital with a serious illness, surrounded by people whose faces you couldn't even see, could not have been easy.

Some people found it difficult to accept. Some refused to go. That meant we had to be at our most persuasive. If all else fails, maybe I could be a double-glazing salesman. We'd tell them how wonderful the nurses were, how they'd make them feel as comfortable as possible. I'd remind them that they could stay in contact with as many people as they wanted, via their phone. It always worked, but they were difficult conversations. And I dare say there were lots of people all over the country who couldn't be persuaded. The only people we left behind were those who didn't need to go to hospital anyway. There were still a lot of people calling 999 when there wasn't much wrong with them.

After the knife attack and recovering from my wobble, I was just glad I wasn't stuck at home like most people. Not least because when I was at home, I suddenly had to become a teacher (unlike the kids of other essential workers, mine didn't go to school). Yes, I've written a book, but I had a bit of help with that. It was like that old Sam Cooke song: 'Don't know much about history, don't know much biology ...' It must have been quite sobering for a lot of parents, discovering that their kids knew more about stuff than they did.

———

Lockdown gave some people time to reflect on their lives, what's important and what isn't. And it meant couples and families could spend a lot more time with each other. But I also wonder what effect it had on some people's mental health. Suddenly, people were cooped up in their houses for weeks on end, often with people they didn't get along with. To make matters worse, they weren't able to access mental health services. People's businesses were falling apart. People were worrying about not being able to pay bills or their rent or their mortgage. Others were suffering in silence with illnesses they'd normally get treated. I knew one chap with terminal cancer whose appointments kept being put back. It's hard to put a figure on how many people the pandemic harmed, besides all those struck down by coronavirus.

As the weeks turned into months, I came to realise that I was in a privileged position. While everyone else was at home, I was still out there helping people. That made me feel more essential than ever. And it wasn't just me. There was a whole army of us – police officers, firefighters, supermarket workers, lorry drivers, carers – carrying on regardless. I felt like a celebrity at times. One time, I was driving down a street in the ambulance and people were all outside clapping. I felt like Lewis Hamilton taking the chequered flag. It was lovely, but I found it a bit embarrassing. I was just doing the job I was paid to do. I don't do that job to get claps, I do it because I have a passion for helping people. Meanwhile, people were losing their livelihoods and their houses. It didn't seem right.

Of course the government made mistakes. They were woefully underprepared for a pandemic and didn't have proper plans in place. The PPE situation was sometimes farcical, and downright dangerous. Our first lot of surgical masks were recalled two weeks later, hearsay on the station was that this was because they were releasing particles that we were then breathing in. The truth we may never know. Then you had the situation with Boris Johnson's chief adviser Dominic Cummings, when he got caught driving to Barnard Castle to 'test his eyesight'. That explanation was an insult to everyone who was staying indoors and abiding by the rules, which was most of the population.

But it was a rapidly changing situation and it's impossible to know if a different government would have dealt with it better. I know a lot of people think that if Boris Johnson had ordered a lockdown earlier, it would have saved a lot of lives. But he couldn't really win and ended up being attacked by all sides. Some people were upset that he wasn't doing enough, others were upset that he was overreacting. I wouldn't have wanted to be in his shoes, that's for certain.

Unsurprisingly, it was a subject a lot of people were very passionate about. As far as I was concerned, and I say this as someone who dealt with the pandemic on the frontline, it was fine to have an opinion that went against the grain. Only a madman would deny that coronavirus was a serious thing that killed thousands of people. The evidence was all around us. But maybe we will look back in a few years' time, when a lot more analysis has been done, and conclude that the cure was worse than the disease. Maybe we'll wonder whether the measures were too heavy-handed, or question why everything was shut down for as long as it was as the economy disintegrated. I'm not saying that's true, but it's a debate that will continue.

What I do know for certain is that coronavirus didn't send us over the edge. We weathered it as a nation and it highlighted just what an incredibly valuable institution the NHS is. Hospitals were strange and foreboding places during the pandemic, even more than normal. Full of apprehension, full of workers speaking muffled words behind masks. But even though you couldn't see their faces, rest assured they were working harder than ever to save lives.

There was, and still is, an awful lot to hate about coronavirus. But I refuse to believe it has created a 'new normal'. I hate that phrase, along with lots of other phrases the pandemic ushered in, which helped spread fear far and wide. This isn't a new normal. There's only one normal, which is what we had before. And we will return to it.

My pride at working for the NHS has never been greater. I hope you feel the same about the NHS, too. And when we do return to the old normal – the real normal – I hope this outpouring of love for the NHS and its workers doesn't ebb away. Because it's that love, above all else, that will sustain it for future generations.

ACKNOWLEDGEMENTS

I would like to thank the folks at Simon & Schuster for giving me the opportunity to write this book, and their subsequent guidance, especially Ian Marshall and Melissa Bond. Thanks to my ghost writer, Ben Dirs, for his passion and commitment in making the scattered parts of an ambulance person's life into a coherent whole. And thanks to my colleagues in the emergency services and NHS for their incredible work and support when things got tough.